RETHINKING PALLI
CARE

A Social Role Valorisation approach

Paul Sinclair

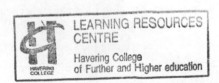

Q

First published in Great Britain in 2007 by

The Policy Press
University of Bristol
Fourth Floor
Beacon House
Queen's Road
Bristol BS8 1QU
UK

Tel +44 (0)117 331 4054
Fax +44 (0)117 331 4093
e-mail tpp-info@bristol.ac.uk
www.policypress.org.uk

© Paul Sinclair 2007

British Library Cataloguing in Publication Data
A catalogue record for this book is available from the British Library.

Library of Congress Cataloging-in-Publication Data
A catalog record for this book has been requested.

ISBN 978 1 86134 921 7 paperback
ISBN 978 1 86134 922 4 hardcover

Cover design by Qube Design Associates, Bristol.
Front cover photograph kindly supplied by Getty Images.
Printed and bound in Great Britain by Hobbs the Printers, Southampton.

For Lisa, Sam, Gabrielle, Matthew, Emily
and my mother

Contents

Acknowledgements

I am indebted to Professor Allan Kellehear for appreciating the value of my insights into palliative care. Without his encouragement, advice and criticism, this book would not have been possible. I would also like to thank him for his support during personal difficulties encountered while writing this book. Lisa Harris has been instrumental in teaching me about Social Role Valorisation (SRV) and the intellectual disability field. I would like to thank her and our family – Sam, Gabrielle, Matthew and Emily – for their love and patience. Sam Sinclair's assistance with cover design has been invaluable. I would like to acknowledge my colleagues at the specialist community-based palliative care service where my ideas took shape. I am also indebted to the many people who used this service for assisting me to reach the perspective contained in this book.

I would also like to thank The Policy Press for their interest and assistance.

List of abbreviations

SRV is used to refer to Social Role Valorisation (Wolfensberger, 1983). This common abbreviation is widely used in intellectual disability services and throughout this book.

PASSING is used to refer to Program Analysis of Service Systems' Implementation of Normalisation Goals (Wolfensberger and Thomas, 1983). PASSING is used in this book to refer to the manual of normalisation measures and criteria for assessing services.

NHWW is used to refer to Nursing Home Without Walls, a service legislated in 1977 in New York State (Miller and Lombardi, 1991).

GP is used to refer to general practitioner.

ONE

Origin of the argument

This book is an argument. And the argument is that palliative care does not deliver on its aims of valuing people who are dying and making death and dying a natural part of life. This book argues for the deinstitutionalisation of palliative care and the development of an alternative framework to institutional approaches, whether these occur in hospices, palliative care units or in community-based palliative care services. This alternative framework consists of a dispersed support network established within the normal communities in which people who are dying live.

This book is original for four reasons. First, no one has previously developed the charge that palliative care fails to deliver on its self-defined mission. Second, no one has previously applied Social Role Valorisation (SRV) (Wolfensberger, 1983, 1998), and the concept of deinstitutionalisation, to the palliative care system. Third, this book is one of the few scholarly contributions that attempts to draw from wider social science perspectives and critically and specifically apply these perspectives to palliative care and its dominant acute care, medical model. Fourth, the conceptualisation of death derived toward the end of this book also breaks new ground, with the reservation that the relevant literature is so vast and complex that there may be some similar drawing together of these ideas of which I am unaware.

Before entering palliative care, I was influenced by the impact of SRV on the intellectual disability service system through my professional and voluntary work with people with an intellectual disability. Moving into the palliative care field, I was struck by the differences between the two systems. Approaches and attitudes that were problematised in intellectual disability services were not considered problems in palliative care. Far from being problems, these same approaches and attitudes were celebrated as ideal in palliative care. That tension created professional dilemmas that became worse with my increasing insight into SRV and palliative care. When I raised these concerns within the palliative care field they were repeatedly rebuffed. It was clear to me that I had to take time to systematise my insights and to clarify the argument.

My concerns were heightened by the fact that my previous

experience with people with an intellectual disability had shown me that a great deal more could be done than I routinely saw being provided in palliative care. I saw not only that more could be done, but that very many things could be done differently. Some people with an intellectual disability with whom I worked had extremely high support needs, including unstable medical conditions. Their needs seemed much greater than anything I ever witnessed in palliative care. Some of these people did not have a familial carer. Nevertheless, year after year, day in day out, 24 hours a day, these people were supported in normal suburban houses. Institutions for people with an intellectual disability had been closed because of the abuse, deprivation and degradation therein. However, institutions in palliative care were believed to be wonderful places, the complete and ideal answer for any eventuality, including eventualities deriving from the social factors that seemed to be behind the vast majority of admissions to institutional care.

Time and again, people were admitted to hospices to die not for clinical reasons but for social ones, yet palliative care activities and programmes and almost all palliative care research were about symptom control, pain management and clinical issues. I could not understand why palliative care was so different from intellectual disability services and yet so similar in other ways. For example, in both areas people who either received support or those who provided it were often called 'special' or 'very special'. If people who were dying were so 'special' I could not understand why the detrimental things I saw happening everyday in palliative care were occurring. To me both fields were about the same thing – living with dignity – irrespective of whether people were living with dying or living with an intellectual disability. It seemed to me that both dying and intellectual disability could be disabling, chronic circumstances. Both were irreversible. Both could require support. And neither dying nor intellectual disability was an illness. Why then did each field use such a contrary approach to the other?

The story *My place* by Sally Morgan (1987), an indigenous Australian, confirmed to me how much more complex and vital the link between identity and place or home is compared to the 'sophisticated' modern view. As a child, I had seen my great aunt and uncle dying in their home. Their dying at home seemed to crown their home and taught me in instinctive ways a deeper appreciation of the meaning of 'my home' and 'my place'. Now as an adult what I saw happening to people who were dying, especially in institutions, made me want to make certain for them a death in their own place, in their own way.

This book is the formal result of those many years of struggle to understand why palliative care is the way it is and those many years of failure to correct the types of injustice I witnessed and perhaps helped perpetrate against people who were dying. It became clear that the mission of the palliative care movement to make death and dying an accepted and valued part of life, which dream I shared in some sense, could never come about by providing palliative care as it was being provided, including by institutionalising people to die. I eventually realised what should have been self-evident from the start.

No valued person chooses to live his/her normal, day-to-day life in institutional care. Therefore, institutional care is self-evidently an abnormal and unnatural way to live. If institutional care is an abnormal and unnatural way to live then, also self-evidently, it must be an abnormal and unnatural way to die, because people live until they die. Since institutional care lies at the heart of the social organisation of palliative care, its influence and its approaches to care must permeate the entire system.

The specific problems for palliative care became clearer when I began using a theoretical framework to analyse various aspects of the palliative care system. In a series of unpublished working papers, I disassembled the entire palliative care system using the lens of SRV theory to discern the original models from which the structures and processes used in palliative care derive. I created a matrix of correspondences between superficially disparate approaches, operating across a range of other fields, and those of palliative care. This work disclosed the almost identical replication of the acute hospital ward system in palliative care. The intrinsic nature of the palliative care system was revealed to be a specialist hospital system with some community outreach. The institution was seen to be the final link in an organisational chain of increasingly restrictive environments of care. In these same working papers, I then reconfigured the palliative care system using SRV theory and the way intellectual disability services were redesigned following deinstitutionalisation. However, from the moment many years earlier that I began applying even a rudimentary understanding of SRV theory to my practice in palliative care, practical ways to ameliorate devaluing effects began to become apparent.

Finally I realised that palliative care itself was one of the most significant factors preventing death and dying from becoming normal, valued parts of life. Palliative care devalued the people it served yet, at the same time, it aimed and claimed to value them. The academic problem became to understand how this contradiction came about and to envision an alternative paradigm for palliative care, based on sound principles that could coherently promote the social valuation of people who are dying.

So the argument presented in this book came about. The book contains three parts: Part One is about the palliative care paradigm. Part Two, about palliative care and social devaluation. Part Three looks at reconceptualising palliative care.

Part One comprises Chapters Two and Three. Chapter Two reviews the past, investigating the historical data concerning the evolution of formal care in general. Modern palliative care did not arise in a vacuum. Palliative care evolved within this larger context of the evolution of formal care patterns. Dominant features clearly appear amid the complexity of developments in formal care from ancient to modern times.

Who provides care? To whom? Why? The answers to questions such as these reveal the broad brushstrokes of the parameters of the paradigm of care. Parameters like 'institutional expression' or 'philanthropic connections' are constant themes, although the specific type of institution or philanthropic connection changes according to the time and place. Particularly with medicine and science supplanting religion in social and political influence in modernity, where once religious institutions and personnel provided care, progressively medical institutions and personnel take over.

Chapter Three examines the ways palliative care reflects or expresses these patterns in the formal development of care in general. This examination shows modern palliative care to conform very closely to the broader paradigm of care. Therefore, the fundamental problems associated with the paradigm of care must also find expression in palliative care. Particularly since the Reformation, the central defect in the conception and organisation of care has been its establishment and propagation of a highly socially valued class of care providers and a highly socially devalued class of care recipients. Only very few received care. The vast majority of the underclass of devalued groups has been excluded from all formal care. This defect was highly functional socially, for example, in 19th-century England the workhouses with their associated infirmaries, where all sorts of devalued groups of people were incarcerated, assured an unending labour force for the industrialising capitalist classes. Since palliative care replicates the paradigm of care, the key problem for palliative care is that it must promote the social devaluation of the people it serves and, as a corollary, must promote the social valuation of palliative care services, sponsors and practitioners.

Part Two consists of Chapters Four and Five and explores the social devaluation of people who are dying as the necessary effect of the current conceptualisation and organisation of palliative care. Chapter Four discusses two alternative frameworks that have informally identified, to some extent, that palliative care is a replication of the late modern form of the paradigm of care by, for example, discerning scientific dualism in core palliative care concepts (Corner and Dunlop, 1997) or by understanding that palliative care is constructed as a medical/nursing discipline (Kellehear, 1998). However, there is no framework that is concerned with the social devaluation of people who are dying, the central defect accompanying this replication, although Kellehear (1990, 1998, 1999) is clearly very aware that social devaluation attends the medical/nursing and medico-psychological models. Since Wolfensberger (1992a, 1998) identifies people who are dying specifically as one of the classes at risk of social devaluation, the argument is made that SRV is the best tool to use to analyse the palliative care system with respect to social devaluation.

Applying SRV theory to palliative care is a complex and massive task since SRV theory can be applied to every level and kind of social interaction. The limited application of SRV theory to palliative care in Chapter Five reveals a general antipathy concerning the negative effects of palliative care services and practitioners, and draws attention to key sources of devaluation by palliative care of people who are dying.

First, the models that underpin palliative care bring with them the devaluation inherent in these models. Second, the devaluation that derives from segregated settings and approaches in palliative care is investigated. Third, the principle to defend valued social roles is applied to palliative care. Fourth, exploring the social imagery conveyed by palliative care shows a deep lack of awareness of the devaluing images in palliative care. Finally, the fundamental belief in the benevolence and necessity of inpatient palliative care facilities is critiqued. This chapter argues that institutional care is not necessary in palliative care. Although problems remain in the intellectual disability services sector, the wholesale dismantling of its vast institutional system is part of the evidence used to support this claim. SRV theory explains that institutional care can never be made benevolent or innocuous because it necessitates the loss of the vast majority of a person's valued social roles. Anything that can be provided in an institution (except an acute care hospital) can be provided in the home, in which case the wholesale elimination of a person's social roles necessitated by institutionalisation can be avoided. The second part of Chapter Five identifies seven paradoxes that are intrinsic to institutional care and institutional approaches to care. These paradoxes expand the broad SRV-based view stated by Wolfensberger (1976a) that the defining characteristic of institutional care is deindividualisation. These paradoxes add further weight to the claim that institutional care can never be 'the answer' and can never be 'fixed'.

SRV theory also describes how to remediate social devaluation. Part Three comprises Chapters Six, Seven and Eight. Chapter Six applies to the palliative care system the same broad structural means used in the intellectual disability services sector to address social devaluation. Institutions take over all responsibility for care and try to provide all relevant services themselves. The way toward the social inclusion of people who are dying must be, therefore, to disperse service provision. The first step entails the closure of palliative care institutions. The second step involves the development of dispersed, non-institutional services, which should occur alongside the closure of institutions. The focus of care cannot shift to the home, the community and the person who is dying while institutions remain.

Chapter Seven seeks to expand the implications of the contradiction between palliative care and its aim to value people who are dying. This disagreement must have some reflection at the philosophical level concerning palliative care's understanding of death. Kellehear's (2005a) ethos of compassion, which is similar to yet more clearly defined theoretically than the palliative care ethos, is used to explore the implications of romantic idealisation concerning the meaning of death. In the process, with the aid of SRV theory, the three faces of death begin to appear as the nature of loss as a universal experience is refined. The triune face of death allows palliative care to connect its romantic idealisation with its modern, mechanistic reductionism regarding the idea of death and to examine the implications of this connection.

The final chapter of the book looks to the future. Since this book is the first formal, scholarly application of SRV to palliative care, other beginning moves in the crossover between SRV and palliative care are described. The future for palliative care cannot be endless repetition of variants of the institutional model. The home should become the centre of the systems of non-acute care. The challenges facing a deinstitutionalised palliative care system are much more straightforward and simple than those that faced the intellectual disability service system. Palliative care should begin the debate that was initiated some 40 years ago in the intellectual disability sector, where currently institutional models are dying but not yet dead, as Taylor (2005) puts it.

This book describes SRV-based shifts away from institutional models of care. These shifts have enabled massive change to occur in the intellectual disability services sector, although the extent to which people with an intellectual disability have managed to gain valued social roles is far from ideal. SRV principles continue to be routinely abused, misapplied and misunderstood by disability services. This book does not mean to imply that the uptake of SRV principles has been uniform or that SRV-based shifts have been able to eradicate the entrenched devaluation in disability services. The social control functions of human services mean that the tendencies toward devaluation will always be present to some degree. This book, therefore, does not intend to imply that the success of SRV-based shifts in the disability sector is by any means complete or unqualified, except concerning the fact that the deinstitutionalised intellectual disability services sector has proven the viability and sustainability of shutting down a vast institutional system.

Although this book contains wide-ranging criticism of palliative care, the author does not intend to deny or dismiss the good faith or good works of palliative care practitioners. Much less does the book intend to imply that practitioners mean to do harmful things to people who are dying. Repeatedly, the book emphasises that palliative care practitioners are, for the most part, unaware of the overarching and pervasive devaluation processes that, it is argued, are intrinsic to the conventional model. This devaluation necessarily, therefore, corrupts current practice. However, the lack of awareness of devaluation processes intensifies the power of these processes by tending to mask their negative effects. The "halo effect" (Flanagan and Holmes, 1999, p 596) surrounding palliative care environments and practitioners also intensifies the power of devaluation for the same reason. This does not mean that nothing good is done. Palliative care's achievements are considerable, as Kellehear (2005a, p 32) notes. The present book does not intend to dismiss or deny these achievements, particularly the reforming of nursing/medical care for people who are dying and the challenging of some of the devaluing social and medical assumptions that underpin hospital maltreatment of people who are dying.

Part One
Palliative care paradigm

TWO

Paradigm of care

Introduction

In this book, the terms 'death' and 'dying' generally denote circumstances other than sudden, accidental, violent or suicidal death. Chapter Seven is the exception since it explores the concept of death itself. The terms 'hospice', 'hospice care' and 'palliative care' are generally used interchangeably. The main exception is when 'hospice' is used to refer to a hospice, an institution, which usage is made clear by the context. 'Palliative care' is used more than 'hospice care' in order to reduce emphasis on the end-stage of dying that is associated with the term 'hospice care'.

In modern times palliative care is one part of a wide-ranging system of care. As a part of the broader social organisation of care in general, the social organisation of palliative care reflects this larger context. An historical analysis of the development of care in general enables palliative care to be set against this broader background. Moreover, if certain patterns of development recur as care has evolved, then these patterns can be used as a framework to analyse the modern social organisation of palliative care.

Patterns in the historical development of care form the template for the kind of social organisation that dominates the modern care system. These patterns also disclose the impact this dominant approach to care has on people who receive care. Through replication of this approach in palliative care, the larger healthcare system imposes itself onto palliative care. Detrimental effects of the care system are thus carried over into palliative care. If palliative care is decontextualised, conceived apart from this broad historical background, then the extent to which it replicates the dominant approach to care cannot easily be established. This opening chapter, therefore, aims to develop a brief historical analysis of the development in western civilisation of the social organisation of care in order to identify the general patterns that recur in this recent palliative care development.

This chapter argues that an overarching paradigm of care can be constructed from this historical analysis. Furthermore, this paradigm consists of features or parameters that constrain the way specific types of care, such as palliative care, are conceptualised. Palliative care literally develops in accordance with these restrictive parameters.

This chapter begins by introducing the key question asked in this book: does palliative care work toward or against its social ideal to make death and dying a natural or normal part of living? The section 'Paradigmatic approach' then examines the main terms of reference for the historical analysis. In this section, an analytical framework is derived from four fundamental questions that generate the four key features or parameters of the paradigm of care. An historical analysis of the paradigm of care begins with, by way of introduction, a brief look at the 'ancient and early medieval (500BC-1050AD) landscape of care' to give some background for later developments. Each of the four key features of the paradigm of care is then explored from the high and late medieval (1050-1550) period through to the modern (1550-2000) period.

Acceptance of death and dying

Does the way we manage palliative care correspond with what we understand death and dying to be? If we understand death and dying to be a normal or natural part of life, to what extent does the social organisation of palliative care reflect this understanding? Smith (1994, p 207) states: "our major challenge is the acceptance of death as a natural part of life, by ourselves, by our patients, by families, and by our culture". In the unanimous opinion of a 1983 study by Rinaldi and Kearl (Kearl, 1989, p 439) of 48 US hospice workers – social workers, directors, coordinators and counsellors – the hospice movement was understood to represent "a general change in social consciousness toward a natural acceptance of death". Hospice care is seen, as one respondent puts it, as "a move toward acceptance of death as a natural part of the life cycle in a culture which has more and more denied the reality that we are mortal" (Kearl, 1989, p 439).

However, the terms 'natural' or 'normal' have no practical meaning outside social context. Normal and natural are synonyms for what is socially valued or socially approved (Conrad and Schneider, 1980). Rumbold (1999, p 64) refers to the "social ideal [of palliative care] to make dying a part of living". Such a statement assumes that currently death and dying are excluded from living or are not a normal part of it or, that is, are socially devalued or disapproved in some sense.

This study is restricted to a consideration of death and dying in western societies. While there is a general view that death and people who are dying are stigmatised (for example, Aries, 1974; Backer et al, 1982, pp 35-9; Kellehear, 1984, p 717; Kearl, 1989, p 443; Field and James, 1993, p 20; Moller, 1996, p 131, with respect to the stigmatisation of the widow and bereavement), the fact of the social devaluation of death and dying remains a matter of debate (for example, Seale, 1998).

While Kellehear's (1990) study does not demonstrate some of the expected characteristics of stigma such as rejection by family, Kellehear asserts that this evidence does not disprove the fact of stigma but rather indicates that its manifestation may be more complex than generally thought. Although favoured, as Seale (1998) notes, as the explanation of the perceived social devaluation of people who are dying, the death-denying society hypothesis is seriously flawed, as both Kellehear (1984) and Seale (1998, pp 52-5) show.

By palliative care returning to the medical mainstream, Rumbold (1999, p 64) contends that palliative care is "now at risk of supporting, not confronting, the denial that keeps death and dying at the margins of society". His solution is to reinvoke the "radical ethos of the hospice movement" via "health promoting palliative care" (Rumbold, 1999, p 66). Such a reassertion of the variably defined original ethos of hospice care is seen as something of a panacea. Bradshaw (1996) sees it as a means to cure, among other things, the ills of professionalisation and humanistic influences in palliative care. Although not mentioning ethos explicitly, Biswas (1993) sees the focus on death and terminal care as that which distinguishes hospice from palliative care, which to her is part of a resurgent medicalisation of hospice care. The original and pristine ethos of hospice care is seen as combating the death-denying society by being somehow death accepting or, in some way, valuing people who are dying in themselves and validating death and the process of dying.

Walter (1991) has also considered societal death denial and the related claim that death is a modern taboo, as suggested originally by Gorer (1965). Kaufmann (1976, pp xvii-xix) argues this claim is ludicrous when at least two generations have tasted death on an unprecedented scale in the 20th century. In addition Kaufmann (1976, pp 219-48) repudiates the entire psychotherapeutic dogma of death denial popularised by Kubler-Ross (1975) that originated with Sigmund Freud's (1915) claim as a psychotherapeutic dictum that "at bottom, no one believes in his own death" (Kaufmann, 1976, p 200). Despite important criticism such as Kaufmann's (1976), the belief in the denial of death became widespread as did the belief in a death-denying society and a death-accepting hospice movement. And so the 'fact' of death denial became observed clinically.

Walter's (1991) discussion helps to clarify the general arguments around the idea of a death-denying society and the social devaluation of death and dying, as does Seale's (1998) discussion. In conclusion Walter (1991, pp 306-7) states that "death [is] highly problematic for the modern individual but not at all problematic for modern society", which "deals with it [death] very nicely thank you by its [modern society's] elevation of youth, education and progress". That is, modern society handles death through making normative those ideals that mask the face and the fact of death. The social relevance of death becomes marginal. The problem of death for the individual is intensified thereby. Mellor (1993) is just one of those who have noted an intensification of the problem of death for the modern individual although he does not attribute this intensification directly to the social values and ideals that are defined as normative. Rather Mellor (1993) favours the related explanation that modern society intensifies the ontological insecurity death represents to individuals by leaving them devoid of frameworks, such as religion, that make sense of death. According to Mellor (1993), death becomes increasingly present in private space and increasingly absent in public space, each process intensifying the other. Clark and Seymour (1999, pp 88-94) provide a summary of the view of death in modernity and in palliative care noting, for example, that "the predominance of good death ideologies can lead directly to the labelling of good and bad patients, and with it the exercise of normative control over the lives of dying people" (Clark and Seymour, 1999, p 93, citing Hart et al, 1998). Under these kinds of analyses, a vicious circle arises. The more society marginalises death's relevance by valuing certain ideals, and not valuing opposing ideals, the greater the problem of death becomes for the individual, and vice versa.

The obverse side of the social valuation of ideals such as youthfulness or progress is the social devaluation of characteristics such as ageing, death and dying that tend to confront or oppose these ideals. This idea at the root of social devaluation has been codified by Wolfensberger (1972, 1992a, 1998). His classifications (Wolfensberger, 1992a, pp 33-4; 1998, pp 9-11) of groups at risk of social devaluation include older people and people with terminal and chronic illness. Wolfensberger (1992a, 1998) derives this classification theoretically by specifying what is highly valued by western society, such as youthfulness and individual independence, and then examining which kinds of people symbolically embody contrary valuations, such as old age and dependence.

By examining the historical landscape of the social organisation of care, of which care for people who are dying is a part, an overview can be gained of the approaches that conform and construct the idea of care. Such an overview can sketch what 'normal', 'good' or socially valued dying and death look like with respect to their social organisation.

Paradigmatic approach

A 'paradigm' (Kuhn, 1962), or 'cosmology' in Jewson's (1976) terms, is a way of seeing or understanding and, more importantly, a way of not seeing. "Cosmologies prescribe the visible and the invisible, the imaginable and the inconceivable. They exclude in the same moment as they include" (Jewson, 1976, p 226). The landscape of the social organisation of the palliative care system discloses the current limits of our imagination in constructing palliative care systems. The palliative care paradigm reveals the possibilities our minds have excluded in the process of creating the present system and, therefore, points to ways to create a more inclusive paradigm.

A paradigmatic approach seeks to view the social organisation of care as a whole. By investigating the historical background of developments in the social organisation of care and the ways in which they are patterned, the paradigm can be seen as a way of including some directions and excluding others. The successful social form is not completely novel but arises out of its antecedent contexts bringing the flavour of these contexts with it. The incremental development of social forms means that developments that are successful have arisen over time through the repeated victory of the ideas and principles that underpin them. These victories necessarily are variously individual, interpersonal, social, political and ideological, as Ramsey (1988) and de Swaan (1990) imply. At times in this incremental developmental process discontinuities appear that represent a novel shift in the paradigm, as Kuhn (1962) demonstrates.

At the same time as successful developments are being validated incrementally, competing developments are being excluded by being invalidated and refuted repeatedly and incrementally. Since a paradigmatic approach seeks to consider the whole landscape, such an approach emphasises firstly, that the appearance of a particular development has excluded alternative ways of social organisation and secondly, that this exclusion discloses patterns or principles in social organisation. A paradigmatic approach to care seeks to reframe conformity to these patterns as the exclusion of difference, of different ways of conceiving, organising and providing care.

Walter's (1991, p 297) criticism of Aries' (1974, 1981) historical study of western attitudes to death raises several weaknesses relevant to the present paradigmatic approach. First, historical evidence accentuates formal rather than informal aspects of care. In spite of this accentuation, "pre-scientific views of the body and disease seem almost ineradicable even in contemporary society" (Ramsey, 1988, p 300). This comment emphasises that formal social development represents the ascendancy of one set of social forms that fit well with the social values and ideals of the time over other sets of social forms and ideas. In acknowledging the debate about the extent to which mental illness itself is socially determined, Porter (1992a, p 301) states "what is beyond dispute, however, is that the strategy of institutionalizing the mad in lunatic asylums [in the 19th century] quite expressly puts into practice many of the key values of Western society since the Renaissance". The present study acknowledges its emphasis on formal patterns of care, although a little attention is given to the informal landscape.

A second weakness concerns the problematic nature of applying modern highly differentiated categories to past eras, as explained by Nutton (1992) and Park (1992). The distinction between formal and informal is problematic except in the highly differentiated social forms of modernity. The meaning of the category 'family' changes, as Herlihy's (1995) discussion illustrates, as does the meaning of 'poor', as Szasz (1994, p 17) notes with respect to the poor as a class. As a final example, the hospital "is coming to be seen as an institution which, though central in modern times [in medical care], need not necessarily be so, and has not necessarily been so" (Granshaw, 1989a, pp 1-2).

In general terms, the weakness of a paradigmatic approach involves the level of simplification and generalisation required to construct a paradigmatic analysis. The diversity of human experience and social development cautions against too rigid a codification of the paradigm of care and implies that a paradigm can only be described with a degree of error. Nevertheless, the value and strength of a paradigmatic approach is that it provides a sense of history, a sense of the contexts out of which successful developments have arisen and a sense of the principles behind the exclusion of alternative developments.

Paradigmatic analysis

Since the social organisation of palliative care occurs within the context of the social organisation of care in general, this paradigmatic analysis, over both Chapters Two and Three, begins by examining the changing paradigm of care. The 'ancient and early medieval (500BC-1050AD) landscape of care' provides a selective initial context to later developments by examining this period under the headings 'medical care' and 'the hospital' since, in later times, these aspects are prominent in the landscape of care.

The chapter then uses the broad answers to four key questions, which are stated shortly, in order to structure the paradigmatic analysis over this chapter and the next. Four key features emerge in answer to these questions and, as a result, these features are used in this chapter to examine the paradigm of care from the high medieval to the modern period.

Each of the four key features and its sub-headings is examined from the high and late medieval period (1050-1550), since as Park (1992, p 75) notes, the beginning of this period marks the start of significant differentiation in the social organisation of medical care from previously relatively undifferentiated forms. The discussion of each sub-heading of each feature continues on to examine developments in the modern period (1550-2000).

The four key features of the paradigm of care are:

- Institutional expression and role system (who provides care to whom? how?)
- Religious ethos (why is care provided?)
- Care of the body, care of the soul (what is cared for?)
- Philanthropic connections (who supports the provision of care? why?)

These key features are divided, with one exception, into sub-headings as follows:

Institutional expression and role system

- Religion and medicine
- Authority, status and respectability
- Social responsibility and social control
- Role system and obligations

Religion and medicine denote the two key institutions concerned with care from antiquity to modernity. Authority, status and respectability attach to religion from antiquity and also to medicine. These institutions express society's responsibility for care and the need to address such things as moral conditions, illness and poverty. To understand the internal functioning of institutions of care, the roles and obligations that operate within and around these facilities need to be explored.

Religious ethos

- Gift of charity
- Morality and meaning

A religious ethos permeates care and Christian culture. Since the gift of Christ's sacrifice out of His charity redeems the Christian, the gift of charity to others by Christians imitates Christ and participates in the act of the redemption of souls. The gift of charity is, therefore, the ideal moral act and is intimately interwoven with the meaning of the suffering of Christ and with the meaning of suffering as such. Significant shifts in these aspects of care occur after the Reformation and again with the secularisation of modernity.

Care of the body, care of the soul

The ancient, inseparable body–soul totality of Christianity becomes split around the 13th century into body and soul (Aries, 1974). With Protestantism, the soul increasingly becomes identified with morality. With modern science and medicine, both the body and mind become compartmentalised into an array of physical and mental components.

Philanthropic connections

- Self-interest
- Privilege versus right

Philanthropy cannot be understood socially and historically as simple charity (Granshaw, 1989a). Self-interest motivates philanthropy to a significant degree. Care is only for a privileged few. The rise of Protestantism shifts the meaning of the privilege of care. With the expansion of modern medicine in the 20th century, care is more of a right now than ever before.

Chapter Three examines the paradigm of palliative care and the problem for palliative care, according to this same scheme, in order to examine how palliative care expresses these key features of the overarching paradigm of care.

Ancient and early medieval (500BC-1050AD) landscape of care

Medical care

Nutton (1992, p 17) indicates that in Greece the popular tradition of self-treatment using herbs stood in contrast to the medical families that became acknowledged within the community as "local medicine men". Because medicine was sacred its knowledge was secret to medical families. Social mobility caused "close intellectual ties" to replace the medical families. Hippocrates (470-377BC) taught anyone "for a fee" (Nutton, 1992, p 19). However, the Hippocratic Oath, which closely resembles the Oath of Freemasonry, formally authorised the secrecy of the closed medical group (Cartwright, 1977, p 41).

The first record of individual physicians dates from the 6th century BC and shows the respect and wealth accorded to doctors (Nutton, 1992, p 19). Broadly speaking, the picture of medical practice was one of a "small group of physicians working alongside lithotomists, midwives and laymen" (Nutton, 1992, p 25).

Religion and medicine existed happily beside each other. Although religious and magical healing were distinguished by doctors, both remained widespread. While both Jew and Christian shared a sense of public duty toward the sick and poor, "pagan concepts of a public duty towards the sick were largely negative", believing the head of the family or a patron should provide support, not the town council or community (Nutton, 1992, p 50). Unlike Greece, doctors in Rome held a relatively low status. Over time, the standing of these doctors improved until the civic doctor became the classical form during the Roman period. "Between the civic doctor and self-help came a great variety of healers – circuit doctors ... wise women, magicians, druggists, faith healers and quacks" (Nutton, 1992, p 53). "The publicly salaried municipal doctor" survived at most up to the 7th century (Park, 1992, p 68). By the early Middle Ages, the majority of medical practitioners were "laymen and women" (Park, 1992, p 69).

The hospital

The first 'hospitals' in the West were temples to Asclepius, the god of healing, in Greece (Cartwright, 1977, p 21), but these were not places where "the sick could reside for long periods under medical supervision" (Nutton, 1992, p 49). Two types of hospitals existed in Roman times: valetudinaria (for slaves and the army) and the private hospitals of the wealthy (closed to the public), for the families of the wealthy (Nutton, 1992, p 50). The slave hospital came into existence because of the decline in the introduction of slaves (Nutton, 1992, p 50), which meant they were no longer as readily replaceable as previously. Eventually, by the early Christian period various types of facility provided care: 'xenodochia' (hospices for pilgrims/travellers), 'nosocomia' (for people who are sick), 'gerocomia' (for older people), 'lobotrophia' (for people with a disability and people with leprosy), 'orphanotrophia' (orphanages) and 'brephotrophia' (foundling homes) (Rosen, 1963, p 4).

In 335AD, all pagan temples including Asclepieia were closed and the "foundation of Christian hospitals followed immediately... In all aspects of disease the Christian emphasis was upon *care* rather than upon *cure*" because "Christianity insisted that disease had a supernatural cause and would only admit a supernatural cure. Thus the devoted care of sick persons tended to express itself in comfort, support and alleviation of symptoms rather than in attempts to deal with the underlying disease" (Cartwright, 1977, p 22; original emphasis).

As the Christian churches became more formalised, so did the social organisation of care. Rosen (1963, pp 3–8) describes the evolution of the hospital under Church directives, which began in 325AD. At first hospitals were established in every cathedral city, and then a 398AD directive required a hospice ('hospitolum'), "very probably" modelled on the pre-Christian "Jewish hospice", to be maintained "not far from the church" (Rosen, 1963, p 3). Although initially small in size, hospitals quickly grew. In the early 9th century, bishops were instructed to establish refuges "for the poor (receptaculum, hospitale pauperum)" (Rosen, 1963, p 7).

"From the ninth century on, monasteries assumed a central role in the care of the poor, and the monastic hospitals became the main institutions serving the needy and the sick, particularly in northern Europe" (Park, 1992, p 71). However, the vast majority of the community relied on "a kind of magic folk-medicine" (Cartwright, 1977, p 11), as Park (1992, pp 64–8) confirms. Local initiatives by some monasteries rather than a "general charitable program" extended care into local communities, especially to the nobility (Park, 1992, p 68). According to Cartwright (1977), the role of monasteries in providing care to the community has been over-emphasised by historians. At the same time, the role of the parish church as community centre, and of the parish priest as untrained medical practitioner, has been under-emphasised (Cartwright, 1977, pp 23–4).

Having provided some selective illustrations of the ancient and early medieval landscape of care, the chapter now examines each key feature of the paradigm of care from the high-late medieval period (1050-1550) through to the modern period (1550-2000), according to the sub-headings previously mentioned (refer 'Paradigmatic analysis' section).

Institutional expression and role system

Religion and medicine

Park (1992) notes that the lack of differentiation in care in the ancient and early medieval period began to change from the 11th century through significant differentiation in medical institutions and practitioners (Park, 1992, p 75). In the early 12th century, the call for monasteries to return to "their original spiritual mission" and away from medical practices "for temporal gain" led to a reduction in secular clergy and monks practising medicine within and outside the monastery (Park, 1992, p 77). As Park (1992, pp 75-82) indicates, despite licensing and standards, unauthorised medical practice remained widespread. Efforts were made to exclude certain groups from medical practice. By 1500, "urban medical practitioners" were "lay, Christian and male (with the exception of midwives)" and "organised to some extent by medical specialty" (Park, 1992, p 81). "An emergent professional culture" was evident (Park, 1992, p 81).

Medicine attained quasi-religious status and function in modernity. The identification of modern medicine as quasi-religious has been confirmed by a large number of authors from many perspectives, for example, Szasz (1961), Halmos (1965), North (1972), Foucault (1973), Illich (1976) and Seale (1998). In antiquity, religion and medicine sat happily together. The modern tension between them reflects the difference in character between the institutional functions of religion traditionally and the quasi-religious institutional functions of medicine in modernity. The supposed moral neutrality of modern medicine sidelines and obfuscates moral issues (Zola, 1977; Conrad and Schneider, 1980). Zola (1972) and Conrad and Schneider (1980) note that deviance, for example, is not removed by medicalisation. Deviance is simply renamed as sickness with its attendant connotations of treatment and curability. As Conrad and Schneider (1980, p 36) state, "disease designation is a moral judgement for to define something as a disease or illness is to deem it undesirable". Conrad and Schneider (1980, p 248) emphasise that this judgement is negative, but that "medical language veils the political and moral fact". According to Zola (1972), the definition of moral action then becomes doing whatever complies with the medical judgement about appropriate responses to the 'illness' (Zola, 1972). Szasz (1994, p 3) states with respect to insanity: "guided by the fake light of compassion, we have subverted the classical liberal conception of man as moral agent, endowed with free will and responsible for his actions, and replaced it with the conception of man as patient, the victim of mental illness".

To the early Church, morality in care meant care for the immortal body–soul totality and an idealisation of the recipients of care. Szasz (1994, p xi) asserts that, in pre-Christian antiquity, care as punishment aimed to improve society not the recipient. Later, in Christian times, referring to St Augustine (354-430), Szasz notes coercion in care was justified as concern to perfect the recipient's soul, not simply to protect society. To the Protestant Church, morality in care meant care for the soul as embodied morality where the moral defect signified by poverty, for example, could be remedied through the moral uplift intrinsic to work. Modern medicine evinces its own morality of care based on the deviant symptom and the body as a collection of parts. The soul has become somatised as the compartmentalised brain or mind. Care of the soul means to diagnose, treat and cure the problems of the mind.

While Zola (1977) emphasises the amoral and asocial character of care under modern medicine, McKnight (1977) asserts that the whole modern human service system emasculates citizens' rights while avowing the apolitical, absolute good of "care" or "love" (McKnight, 1977, p 72). The difficult moral issues of determining what behaviours should be treated and in what directions, which are noted by Conrad and Schneider (1980, p 276) citing Wootton (1963), are excluded by modern medicine's supposed moral neutrality and physical reductionism. The further moral issues concerning "what freedom should an individual have over his/her body, or what else, beside the individual, needs treating", which are noted by Zola (1977, p 64), are also excluded.

In the modern period, the central value dichotomy moves away from a religious or moral basis, shifting from what is or is not good, to what is or is not rational (Porter, 1992a, p 301). Szasz (1994, pp xi-xii) describes this as a shift from the theological to the therapeutic state. Medicine not religion began to define what was deviant, and did so increasingly. For example, the social devaluation of the insane was accelerated by their institutionalisation (Porter, 1992a, p 282). 'The mad' were not considered a threat, as Porter (1992a) notes in respect of the 18th century, and insanity not considered primarily a 'moral category', as Park (1992) notes in respect of the late Middle Ages. Incarceration in medical institutions served, therefore, not only to accelerate but also to institutionalise the social devaluation of insanity that persists to this day despite its relabelling as sickness. Conrad and Schneider (1980) give several further examples of the modern medicalisation of deviance.

Authority, status and respectability

The idea of 'informal care' in ancient times needs to be understood in the context of the family. In antiquity the idea of family was one that applied only to the elite because the vast majority of people were either very poor or slaves (Herlihy, 1995, p 138). With the establishment of the family at all levels of society by about the end of the Middle Ages, more for the rich than for the poor, the role of women in informal care could expand because the role of women in formal social and economic roles became restricted. From this time the differentiation of informal care by women both in the home and in the community became discernible. Herlihy (1995, p 138) notes the female role of the "practice of charity". However, the historical landscape of informal care is far from clear even with respect to the role of the family around the deathbed. Porter's claim (cited in Houlbrooke, 1998, p 219) that in the 18th century the family became absolutely central to the deathbed scene is questioned by Houlbrooke (1998, p 219), who finds bias in the evidence. Houlbrooke (1998) asserts that the family had always played a central role at the deathbed (at least from the 15th century in which his study begins). He explains that family involvement is found less in the evidence because it was considered unremarkable relative to the religious aspects of the deathbed. However, later in the secularising 18th century the reduced religious focus increased the relative significance of the family's deathbed role. Kellehear (2005a) provides an account of the history of informal or community care.

Medieval hospitals were "houses of religion" (Orme and Webster, 1995, p 35), with the authority, status and respectability attending the Church. From the mid-13th century, specialised institutions concerned with public health were developed (Park, 1992, p 83). The hospital for the sick poor founded by Christians was the major institutional development of the medieval period. The hospital spread not only because of Church initiatives but "because it became a central institution around which great hospital and nursing orders established themselves" (Rosen, 1963, p 7), such as the Knights Hospitaller of St John (1099). In the early 14th century, some of such orders' foundations excluded "incurables", that is "the chronically ill" (Park, 1992, p 89) who were the traditional clientele, to focus on "the acutely ill" and sometimes also "children and pregnant women" (Park, 1992, p 85). A routine medical presence in hospitals, along with other practitioners, was evident in 15th-century Italy (Park, 1992). A beginning medical presence was evident in English hospitals only from the 16th century (Carlin, 1989, p 30). The plague, in 1348 and recurrently until the end of the 15th century, cemented the shift in the purpose of hospitals from charity to public health (Park, 1992, p 87). Hospitals increasingly admitted only the acutely ill. Incurables and the chronically ill poor were excluded from hospitals for a complex range of reasons. The 15th century saw large institutions for specific groups of the chronically ill, such as the blind and the insane, begin to be established. For example, the English hospital St Mary of Bethlehem (1247), the infamous Bedlam, wholly specialised in the care of insanity by the mid-15th century (Cartwright, 1977, p 31; Park, 1992, p 89).

Returning to 'informal care', in the medieval and early modern period a "comprehensive lay medical culture" was "rooted in the community and its wisdom" and operated within a web of social expectations and obligations (Porter, 1992b, p 97). By the late 18th century general practitioners were numerous in England. Voluntary hospitals and outpatient dispensaries had proliferated (Porter, 1992b, p 100). Professional medicine was much more available to greater proportions of the population (Porter, 1992b, p 100). "Amongst the more affluent classes and in the new lying-in hospitals for the poor, male accoucheurs replaced traditional midwives and the community rituals of giving birth" (Porter, 1992b, p 101). Other outcomes of this medicalisation were a "decline of magical medicine and the marginalisation of wise women and cunning men" (Porter, 1992b, p 100). The "public or private lunatic asylum often presided over by a regular medical man" replaced the home or some form of parish care for the insane and granted "the practitioner a heroic role" (Porter, 1992b, p 101). However, in the 18th century this initial stage of medicalisation did not "erode routine self-medication or the lay health culture at large", but rather sought "to co-opt" and "control it" (Porter, 1992b, p 101).

These developments illustrate the tendency for a professionalised model of medicine with significant institutional expression to seek to exclude alternative models of care and absorb their markets. At this stage, the dominant power of the patient in the doctor–patient relationship meant this attempt was frustrated, leaving doctors to endlessly describe the consequences of disobedient patients and obsessive self-diagnosis (Porter, 1992b).

Women, and particularly those without formal training, progressively were shifted out of formal care (Addams, 1993). Addams' (1993) early 20th-century picture of a team of women, led by an older more experienced woman, assisting in the home with a broad range of supportive and 'professional' roles in any area of need, especially birth and death, may be typical of long-standing patterns of informal care in Anglo-Saxon communities. The similar example noted by Addams (1993, p 158) adds weight to this possibility. Kellehear (2005a) notes the takeover of community care by professionals during the past 150 years.

In suggesting that the ideas of home care and hospice existed more than 200 years ago, Backer et al (1982, p 50) note that in the 18th century many still "believed the home was the only possible place for recovery" because of "all the natural curative and caring aspects of family life – the benevolence, the comfort, the consolation". These authors also claim this set-up had the added benefits of reducing national costs and minimising the spread of infection. Although this picture is simplified, it is certain that for a long time hospitals (for the sick poor) were identified with pauperism and death (Granshaw, 1989a, p 1) whereas almshouses, even in the 20th century, could provide the privilege of residential care into a long old age (Bailey, 1988, pp 197-9). In noting unfillable vacancies in those almshouses run by the Church in Britain in the 1980s, Bailey (1988, p 195) explains this might be due to the deterrent effect of "restrictions of movement, compulsory religious services, and other rules and regulations – not to mention qualifications for entry". That these kinds of demands still exist, after many centuries, points to their centrality within the paradigm of care and supports the view that this kind of servility strongly influences the notion of compliance in medical settings.

With respect to more formal aspects of care, the reason for the ongoing expansion of voluntary hospitals or infirmaries lay in the need for the capitalist class to delude the poor through "elaborate and spectacular rituals of paternalistic care" (Porter, 1989, p 152). "Unlike the hospices and the earlier hospitals, these 'new' hospitals were not for paupers but for the industrious poor and, in particular, for the urban poor" (Maggs, 1987, p 178). By the mid-18th century medical practitioners were wealthy enough to afford to donate their services to infirmaries so as to seek the status of gentlemen (Porter, 1989, pp 159-61). This is the origin of the consultant's honorary status. Most of these consultants' wealth came from their very lucrative private practices to the wealthy, which involved the practice of medicine and surgery but rarely that of pharmacy and midwifery (Waddington, 1977, p 170). However, hospital teaching and the apprenticeship of student surgeons were also very financially rewarding (Waddington, 1977, p 170). These arrangements ensured that only the most respectable could enter the medical elite. Another important effect of this elite closed shop was that hospital medical staff became known (to private patients) as possessing the most advanced expertise (Abel-Smith, cited in Waddington, 1977, p 171).

Throughout the 18th and 19th centuries, the 'economies of scale' argument "runs like a watermark through the propaganda of the voluntary hospitals" (Porter, 1989, p 163). This economy was conditional. Those who required chronic, terminal or infectious care were excluded by 'medical screening' and the non-deserving poor were excluded through the 'private screening of subscriber nomination' of inmates (Porter, 1989).

Power began to shift in the early 19th century in the medical institution from private benefactors to medical men due in part to the repercussions of the new medical gaze characterised by Foucault (1973, p 89) as: institutionally validating and endorsing the doctor as the agent with "the power of decision-making and intervention ... always receptive to the deviant [sign/symptom]" and capable of calculating risks. Following Foucault, Backer et al (1982) state that teaching and research functions characterise the uniqueness of the modern hospital.

The modern hospital structure enabled the medical closed shop to develop through training its members and conducting research. The development of the psychiatric closed shop further supports this view. Porter (1992a, p 289) describes the private lunatic asylum as the "formative site for the development of psychiatry" through research on large numbers of 'mad' people collected together. Anleu (1995, p 147) concurs: "the separation of deviants was an essential pre-condition for the development of a medical specialty (the forerunner of psychiatry) claiming to possess a specific expertise to deal with madness". Collecting people, whose primary similarity lies in their illness, condition or, that is, their deviance, together in an institution not only facilitates the professionalisation of the provider group, by developing a specialised body of knowledge, but also reflects and deepens the deviance of the class of people with the condition.

By the end of the 19th century, cure of disease had replaced the holistic medieval conception of care (Granshaw, 1989b). The 19th century saw a rapid expansion of hospitals throughout the West. Although the emphasis on disease classification was increasing, hospitals had for some time been specialising in various conditions because it was a way to generate both income and status for medical practitioners (Granshaw, 1989b). The management of lunacy was shifted out of poor relief by the new Poor Law (1834). From that point, the management of lunacy was able to become increasingly under medical control (Cummins, 1968). In explaining that the movement to medicalise US asylums around the turn of the 20th century was a reform movement based on the idea of cure, Church (1987, pp 109-10) quotes Cowles (1887): "'attendants' may attend the infirm and incurable, but 'nurses' attend the sick, and the experience of recovery from illness is so common that the very presence of a nurse logically carries with it the other idea, that something is being done to promote recovery, and that in itself inspires hope and is curative". This statement captures the archetypal symbolism of the nurse and illness (and, by implication, the doctor) and indicates that the significance of the images of medical authority has been well understood and utilised for some time. Just as the medical specialty, gerontology, validates and signifies the existence of the illness of ageing (Zola, 1977), so too the existence of the new medical specialty, palliative medicine, validates and signifies the existence of the illness of dying. Medical images signify illness and its cure or eradication and the hope attaching to this cure or eradication.

The development of specialist hospitals helped place the doctor at the centre of medical care (Granshaw, 1989a, p 10). Specialist hospitals used the methods of the general hospital medical men before them to achieve status, authority and respectability. Outpatient dispensaries, well developed by the late 18th century (Granshaw, 1992), had no value for this purpose. In the 19th century, therefore, specialised outpatient dispensaries were replaced by specialist inpatient hospitals (Granshaw, 1989b, p 202; Seidler, 1989, p 184). The medical establishment loudly proclaimed specialist hospitals to be improper and inferior (Granshaw, 1989b). The preservation of economic and social privilege motivates the medical elite's rage against the specialist hospital and outpatient and community care.

A threatened market and the threat to the general hospital as the repository of the ultimate expertise drove the medical establishment to compete resolutely with the specialist hospitals. From around 1864, general hospitals in England began appointing their own specialists to undermine specialist hospitals until the victory of the general hospital in 1948 when the National Health Service "took at face value the criticisms [by general hospitals and the medical establishment] of specialist hospitals" (Granshaw, 1989b, pp 209, 215).

The specialist cancer hospitals eventually went the same way as other specialist hospitals before them. General hospitals absorbed specialist hospitals. Although specialist hospitals were responsible for considerable progress in medicine, they dishonestly proclaimed their purpose as the advancement of medical science when, as has been mentioned, their purpose concerned improving the status of doctors. Specialist cancer hospitals were not founded to advance medicine but rather to emphasise the religious, medieval idea of hospice (Murphy, 1989, p 221). The Irish Sisters of Charity, whose mission was to serve the sick poor, had cared for the sick in their homes until in 1879 their first specialist institution of care for people who were dying was opened in Dublin (O'Leary, 1988). Wolfensberger (1984, p 168) suggests some similarity between St Christopher's Hospice and the seven homes for the dying operated by the Hawthorne Dominican Sisters/Servants whose work began in 1896 and continues to this day in the US. Toward the end of the 19th century, cancer hospitals in England had plans for homes for people who were dying, but this idea was shelved by them for the better part of a century until the modern hospice movement came into being. (Clark and Seymour, 1999, and Clark, nd, provide further detail and references regarding the antecedents of hospice care.)

General hospitals refused to take patients with advanced cancer and dying charity patients had always been turned away from general pauper infirmaries (Murphy, 1989). Almost all cancer hospitals that did not adopt the new scientific approach did not survive beyond the 19th century (Murphy, 1989). Cancer hospitals decreasingly cared for dying patients (Murphy, 1989). It was well understood that money would be readily available from the philanthropic and community sectors to support the efforts of the medical profession's research into a cancer cure rather than to the low status care for people who were dying (Murphy, 1989). The capacity to access formal care, and the quality and type of care once it is accessed, is related to the social value of the recipient of care. 'Incurables' when they had been idealised could receive institutional care. In late medieval times, the curable became the favoured clientele for hospitals, even such as those of the Hospitaller Orders with a traditional commitment to 'the incurable'. In modernity, with the demonisation of the pauper and the ascendancy of the idea of cure, 'incurables' became an unwanted class. Common 'incurables', that is those not benefactor/subscriber nominated, have been excluded from institutional care from at least the late Middle Ages until the early part of the 20th century. In the mid-17th century insanity was regarded as incurable. The confinement of the insane in asylums over the next century and a half accompanied the change in belief that insanity could be cured (Porter, 1992a). The idea of cure or treatment tends to be accompanied by some form of institutionalisation of the class of people thought to have the relevant condition. The pattern of absorption and colonisation of alternative approaches to care continued with the specialist cancer hospital.

In late modernity, every condition, every behaviour has become amenable to medical and/or medico-psychological treatment, at least potentially, and amenable to medical and/or medico-psychological cure, at least potentially. Within this framework, alternative medicine, self-medication and complementary therapies have become the new face of the resilient and adaptable lay medical culture and pre-scientific ideas about illness. The prerogative to prescribe, however, has remained a medical monopoly. Anleu (1995, p 145) asserts that "medical dominance and autonomy remain largely intact, especially as one of the profession's responses to competition from complementary health practitioners is to incorporate elements of non-medical, social welfare or holistic health into its own practice while simultaneously excluding alternative practitioners".

Authority, status and respectability attend both the hospital and the medical profession. The exclusion of competing practitioners by the medical elite and its hospital, while at the same time colonising their markets, has a long history. Status differentials within the medical profession ensured the preservation of the hospital as the scholarly repository of the highest medical expertise, notwithstanding the victory of the general practitioner (GP) for inclusion within the medical elite. Medical practitioners in England in the 17th century have traditionally been divided into three groups. First on the list came university-educated physicians, who were of much higher status than surgeons, the second type of practitioner. The third group, the apothecaries, were of similar status to surgeons (Porter, 1992b, p 93). Predominantly only the affluent could access these services. The apothecary's role overlapped both the physician's and the surgeon's. By the 18th century, the surgeon-apothecary is established, the prototype of the GP (Porter, 1992b, pp 92-3). By the early 19th century the GP had arrived, the "combined man midwife and surgeon-apothecary" (Loudon, 1992, p 233). GPs' low competence and low social status, which derived from them treating the poor, from GPs' low income and from their practice of pharmacy, was underscored by the denigration received from the medical elite (Loudon, 1992, p 242). Finally, adopting a combined pastoral and clinical role, the "family doctor" arrived by the mid 19th century (Loudon, 1992, p 243).

Without the conflict between the medical elite and GPs, the eventual rise in GP status "could have meant a system of education based on training in the community rather than hospitals with a greater emphasis on the common diseases and the problems of public health" (Loudon, 1992, p 245). The medical reform beginning in the late 18th century was caused by the struggle for "rank, title and status, linked to questions of social and professional respectability, which in turn were linked to questions of fees and income" (Loudon, 1992, p 229). GPs sought social respectability in the same way physicians had. The incorporation of GPs, and so their markets, into the medical elite with its central dependence on the hospital meant that the community and social focus of medicine was able to be colonised by the new medical establishment. Alternative models that might not have placed the hospital at the centre of the system of care were excluded.

Similar concerns have been raised with regard to nursing. Maggs (1987) refers to Carpenter (1980) in noting that branches of nursing care other than general hospital nursing receive little attention from historians of nursing. Maggs (1987, p 4) states that "in this way historians confirm, rather than question, the dominance of hospital nursing in the constellation of nursing and nursing-linked occupations". The ascendancy of general hospital nursing occurred at the expense of a variety of other groups and organisations (Maggs, 1987, p 5). The tendency for the hospital-centred model of care to absorb or exclude alternative forms of nursing care is evident when Krampitz (1987, p 89) emphasises the value of the lessons to be learned from nursing history concerning the medical system since, in the 1980s, "nurses must again make a concerted effort to move from the hospital into community-based professional practice".

The most important late 20th-century challenge to medicine has come from the state seeking to "curb the autonomy of the medical profession" (Lewis, 1992, p 342). Moves toward preventative medicine, health promotion, community care and the "Cinderella specialties such as geriatrics and psychiatry" have been pushed by the state to try to shift funds from the acute sector supported by the medical profession (Lewis, 1992, p 342). Palliative care can be seen as another such Cinderella specialty. In Britain, consumer empowerment, centralisation and an entrepreneurial delivery system have been seen as the state attempting to master medical professional power (Lewis, 1992).

Social responsibility and social control

The medieval period showed that "a system of relief is little more than the succour which the 'haves' are agreed and willing to provide to the 'have nots'" (Rubin, 1989, p 57), generally for the purpose of "personal and collective gratification and in order to promote the stability and order of their communities" (Rubin, 1989, p 56). Medieval English hospitals ('hospitale') consisted of four main types:

- the most numerous almshouses for 'the poor', older people or local community members and/or others specially prescribed by benefactors (Carlin, 1989, p 24; Henderson, 1989, p 63);
- the lazar houses (for leprosy);
- the least numerous infirmaries, founded by monasteries, for 'the sick poor' (Carlin, 1989, p 21); and
- the hospices for travellers/pilgrims (Bailey, 1988, p 16; Carlin, 1989, p 21).

The main functions of the hospitals were worship, charity to the poor, sick and travellers, and education and learning (Orme and Webster, 1995, pp 49-68). Charity was divided into four types: "long-term maintenance of the infirm, medium-term care of the sick until they should recover, short-term hospitality to travellers, and regular distribution of alms to the poor", with many hospitals specialising in certain of these functions (Orme and Webster, 1995, pp 57-8).

However, in the latter part of the 14th century an emergent differentiation in hospitals' purpose became apparent to combat increasing vagrancy (Cartwright, 1977, p 30). From the 14th century care of the sick became an impossible task for most medieval hospitals because of the numbers who needed care (Carlin, 1989, p 25). As this problem worsened, together with the post-Reformation attitude that the poor were indolent if not evil, the burden of the sick and poor became unwelcome. Increasingly the hospital as an institution of social control became accentuated.

The key development of the 16th century was the Dissolution between 1536-47 of the monasteries, hospitals and guilds. As well as the financial abuse in hospitals, vagrants were increasingly using relief intended for the sick and aged. Only a few almshouses remained (Cartwright, 1977, p 33). The state exercised increasing control over the poor. The deserving and undeserving poor were first distinguished in 1563 (Parsons, 2004). However, in questioning the view that this discrimination originated in the 15th and 16th centuries, Orme and Webster (1995, p 57) imply an age-old aspect to devaluing attitudes despite idealisation of the "indigent and sick as images of Christ". "From the first, people approved of some poor, disapproved of others, a discrimination bound to affect the working of hospitals which were also run by human beings" (Orme and Webster, 1995, p 57). The Poor Law (1601) initiated the state's first formal role in welfare. The poor were punished increasingly after the Reformation, which demonised them as a "source of sedition, crime and disease, to say nothing of witchcraft" (Bailey, 1988, p 87). Poor relief was therefore as much a "matter of state security as of pity" (Bailey, 1988, p 87).

Early in the 15th century rather than institutional care such as St Mary of Bethlehem, the Belgian town of Geel with its healing shrine to St Dymphna developed an alternative type of care for the insane centred on home care (Park, 1992, pp 89-90). Dumont (1994) indicates that the Geel community integrated the possessed/insane into their daily living. Citing his own 1962 study, Dumont states: "in Geel ... where patients are almost entirely unrestrained and where the tolerance of deviant behaviour in the community is extraordinarily high, schizophrenia does not appear to be a very disabling disease" (Dumont, 1994, p 38). Commenting that religious idealisation of a class of people has some power to resist institutionalisation of that class, Wolfensberger (1972, p 72) describes several examples, including Geel, where the religiously idealised often child-like role imposed on people with an intellectual disability has given rise to non-institutional models of care. Familiar changes occur in Geel's care system.

> The family care system in Geel was supervised by the local municipality until the Ministry of Justice took over in 1850.... In 1861 an infirmary was built ... inspired by Dr Guislain's progressive ideas on the treatment of mental illness.... It wasn't until 1948 [that] the family care programme came under the supervision of the Ministry of Public Health and Welfare (OPZ Geel, 2006, History).

Following the Reformation in England, significantly increased numbers of old, sick and unemployed people died on the streets "without mercy" (Bailey, 1988, p 87). The tremendous punishments for poverty, which began at the start of the 16th century, peaked around the beginning of the 18th century when the "penalty for stealing a loaf of bread to ward off starvation was death by hanging" (Bailey, 1988, p 141). The workhouse system with its associated infirmaries came into being in England with the new Poor Law of 1834 (Crowther, 1981; Bailey, 1988, p 141). As Bailey states: "the workhouse was the logical tool of the doctrine that any handout to the genuinely poor should be accompanied by penalties" (Bailey, 1988, p 141). The poor would be institutionalised en masse and forced to work, even if only a fraction of them were able-bodied.

Systematic institutionalisation of the poor from 1834 was the final solution to their demonisation. Szasz (1994, p 17) comments that a 1714 law required authorised lunatics to be kept in parish-erected Bridewells (a precursor of the workhouse and named after the London penitentiary near St Bride's Well). These degenerated into 'receptacles of misery' for all types of unwanted people. The infamous history of the workhouse system and the asylum demonstrate that institutionalisation of a specific category of people tends to reflect, validate, accelerate and intensify the social devaluation of that class.

In the 17th century the idea of specialised institutional management for various groups simultaneously began to take root (Park, 1992), of which the hospital solely for the sick was one. The most dramatic phenomenon, however, is the 'great confinement' of the mad (and others), as Foucault (1988) termed it. Porter (1992a) and Park (1992) qualify significantly Foucault's account, Park (1992, p 90) noting that it was punitive attitudes to "chronically ill indigents" that developed rather than such attitudes to the insane specifically. Although "insanity had never been primarily a moral category ... unlike leprosy" (Park, 1992, p 88), it was considered shameful because of "overtones of either diabolical possession or of hereditary taint" (Porter, 1992a, p 279). The incorporation of 'the mad' in normal medieval hospitals until the period of the asylums supports this contention (Porter, 1992a). Before the mid-17th century, 'the mad' had been periodically ejected from towns via ships, for example (Anleu, 1995). Evidently, 'the mad' were socially devalued but not morally toxic.

Whereas once 'mad' people had been cared for informally at home or under some type of parish care, institutionalisation of 'the mad' began at least from the mid-19th century in private asylums (Porter, 1992a, pp 281-92). Just as there was money to be made from providing medical care to the wealthy, there was money to be made from caring for madness among the wealthy. The 'trade in lunacy' (Parry-Jones, 1972) was lucrative and saw the establishment in the 17th century of numerous private asylums. These asylums also housed unwanted and troublesome sane members of wealthy families (Porter, 1992a, p 284). Following the Industrial Revolution, the number of medical hospitals grew dramatically, as did both large and small lunatic asylums. By the end of the 18th century the medical model of madness under the control of physicians was dominant (Anleu, 1995, p 146). The massive growth in both the numbers of asylums and the numbers of inmates occurred in the 19th century when asylums became the dumping grounds for all kinds of socially devalued people.

In the mid-19th century, Howe (1976, p 33) states:

> ... idiots form one of that fearful host which is ever pressing upon society with its suffering, its miseries, and its crimes, and which society is ever trying to hold off at arm's length, – to keep in quarantine, to shut up in jails and almshouses, or, at least, to treat as a pariah caste; but all in vain.

At that time, Howe helped introduce in the US the system of special schools for various groups including people with an intellectual disability, which system was adopted "throughout Europe and the US" (Ferleger and Boyd, 1980, p 166). Wolfensberger (1975, p 17) asserts that Howe "had already perceived and accurately defined most of the shortcomings under which institutions would labour for the next 100 years". Although initially much more humane than existing institutional options, "the schools of the mid-1800s became the institutions of the mid-1900s [in the US]" (Ferleger and Boyd, 1980, p 166). In 1900, in the US, these institutions "resembled a small town" (Heal et al, 1980, p 217). If for no other reason than the categories making up the 'fearful host' of the deviant were not well defined, institutions for a certain group incarcerated a variety of deviant classes into the mid-20th century.

Medicine has assumed the fundamental social control role in late modernity (Zola, 1972, 1977). Professionalisation, especially when this profession is centred on an institution, is linked to social control. In the 20th century, the 'expropriation of health' (Illich, 1976) by the medical industry has also become an expropriation of life (Zola, 1972). All of life has become a medical and medico-psychological concern, at least potentially. The mid-20th century "psychiatrization of everything" (Porter, 2002, p 199) is reflected in a rapidly expanding psychiatric taxonomy, which exhibits "wholesale comings and goings of disease classifications" with each subsequent edition of the *Diagnostic and statistical manual of mental disorders* (Porter, 2002, p 216). The "psychiatrization of everything" has created and is fed by an ever-expanding "victim culture" (Porter, 2002, p 217), where "more are said to be suffering – indeed more are *claiming* to be suffering – from a proliferation of psychiatric syndromes" (Porter, 2002, p 217; original emphasis). The World Health Organisation's Ottawa Charter (1986) defines health holistically as "an empowered lifestyle which is more than merely absence of illness" (Kellehear, 1998, p 4). This extension of what health is defined to be tends to collude with and further authorise the medicalisation of life as an idea.

Role system and obligations

The earliest English hospitals were modelled on religious institutions (Rubin, 1989, p 44). A monastic community translated readily to the idea of the religio-therapeutic hospital community where a religious vocation and role structure served the religious mission. "The organisation and administration of a lay hospital was very similar to that of a monastic infirmary" (Cartwright, 1977, p 24).

Many hospitals were cruciform in shape like a church (Cartwright, 1977, p 24; Bailey, 1988). The chapel, the central station, enabled surveillance (Murphy, 1989, p 76). In late-medieval and Renaissance Florentine hospitals, the altar, the central station, both enabled surveillance by medical staff and allowed patients to see Mass being celebrated (Henderson, 1989, p 76). Monastic rules or strict obligations, even sometimes including robed dress, were applied to hospital inmates (Bailey, 1988). The role of the person in institutional care might best be described as one of gratitude through servility. Often formal founder-worship was required. Punishments accompanied even very minor infringements of the rules (Bailey, 1988).

Until the 19th century, doctors had to prove their gentlemanliness to be retained, rather than any skill, because doctors held inferior social status to their patients (Waddington, 1973, p 213). In the (Paris) hospitals, the doctor first became the dominant member in the doctor–patient relationship (Waddington, 1973, pp 213-14). The right to consent and to privacy of the body were able to be abused within the hospital setting. Generally, only the poor and those without support attended hospitals because large numbers of people died from cross-infection in the unsanitary conditions of hospitals (Waddington, 1973). If poor patients refused treatment, or created even "the slightest difficulty" (Waddington, 1973, p 216), they were discharged immediately. In this environment dreadful experimentation took place, so that medical knowledge could expand (Waddington, 1973). Burdens of charity also could not refuse to be observed while undergoing treatment. Medical practitioners' expropriation of power set the precedent for a similar expropriation by the whole professionalised human service system in the 20th century. Even throughout the 18th century publicly displayed inmate gratitude was still an obligatory role (Porter, 1989, p 168).

Religious ethos

Gift of charity

Medieval hospitals were regarded as spiritual foundations belonging to the jurisdiction of the Church (Orme and Webster, 1995, p 32). The religious ethos permeated the very idea of hospital.

From the early Christian period, the poor/sick inmate's poverty/ sickness was idealised as a virtue (Bailey, 1988, p 104) by an inversion of values supported, for example, by the Biblical injunction that the first shall be last and in the very old prayer of dedication of the Knights Hospitaller of the Order of St John (Order of Malta, 1992). This idealisation was eroded post-Reformation, although it still exists strongly in Catholicism. In this inversion of values, the recipients of care, as embodiments of Christ, represent an opportunity for such orders to participate in the redemptive act via charity. The L'Arche communities of France for people with an intellectual disability are another modern example of a similar value inversion (Bayley, 1991, pp 92-3). These communities are also a clear example of the Christian religious ethos of care. This ethos centres on valuing recipients of care in themselves, or valuing them for what they can teach others, including care providers, about themselves in a spiritual sense (Bayley, 1991, pp 89-94). Idealisation of the recipients of care is a fundamental feature of the religious ethos.

In the early modern period, hospitals continued to be modelled on religious institutions in name as well as in structure and ethos. Religion continued to be used to promote respectability and authority. For example a saint's name, "any saint's name", for a specialist hospital was used to confer status to medical men and the institution (Granshaw, 1989b, p 205), as already obtained with voluntary hospitals. Some English hospices are now located in old hospitals. Palliative care, therefore, has inherited, at least in England, some of the aura from the many hospitals 'sanctified' in this way. The voluntary hospitals or infirmaries embodied the idea of care as charity and a privileged gift. Braudel's term "gift relationship – he who gives dominates" (cited in Granshaw, 1989a, p 8) is used by Porter (1989, p 150) to characterise the philanthropic motive behind the establishment of the voluntary hospitals. This 'gift relation' (Porter, 1989) is fundamentally interwoven with the idea of charity.

The religious ideal of charity and its religious ethos were in the 19th century to be reformalised in nursing, both in hospitals and in community care. In 1889, the Kansas visiting nursing association, whose developmental "history was replicated across the US", originated as a "small-scale philanthropic religious endeavour" (Lineback, 1987, p 140). District nurses were established in England and trained from 1857 by Florence Nightingale and her colleague Sister Mary Jones (Cartwright, 1977, pp 156-7). The latter was a member of the Anglican nursing sisterhoods. Nightingale also worked with Mary Aikenhead (1787-1858) the founder of the Irish Sisters of Charity (Murphy, 1989, p 235), who were also influential at this time providing domiciliary nursing as well as inpatient care. According to Bradshaw (1996), Nightingale's revivalist faith was also influenced by her training with the Lutheran nursing order at Kaiserswerth in Germany. Nightingale became convinced that an independent sisterhood was the way to secure hospital reform and make female nursing a paid occupation (Cartwright, 1977, p 155; Godden, 1997, p 177). To this end, Nightingale "utilised images of the nurse, not as a paid worker, but as a quasi-religious, ladylike philanthropist" (Godden, 1997, p 177) and "increasingly exploited religious and philanthropic ideals" (Godden, 1997, p 186). Modern professional nursing is rooted in the ethos of the religious sisterhoods.

By the end of the 19th century the professionalisation of social work was well underway in the UK with Octavia Hill and then a little later in the US with Mary Richmond. Naturally the antecedents of social work in charitable work brought a strong religious ethos of charity and service to the poor into the new profession. This religious flavour to social work remained strong despite secularisation through professionalisation.

Morality and meaning

A Catholic-dominated context where the poor were idealised was modified by the Protestant context that was suspicious of the other-worldly mechanisms of Catholicism such as the idea of intercession by the saints, whose relics played a central role in the management of the dead, as Aries (1981) indicates. Protestantism doubted an ongoing relationship between the living and the dead with complex repercussions for the meaning of suffering, purgation and death. Prior (1989, p 167) remarks that still, in modern Ireland, the ongoing active relationship between the living and the dead of the Catholic decisively contrasts with the Protestant way.

With the shift to demonisation of the poor, and to their uplift through the moral integrity of work, the morality behind care changed. A similar shift was evident in attitudes to intellectual disability. "In ancient

Greece and Rome the mentally handicapped were treated as objects of scorn and persecution" (Rosen et al, 1976, p xiii). With Christianity came pity for people with an intellectual disability, and then in medieval times some retained some value as "jesters and fools" (Rosen et al, 1976, p xiii). However, both "Luther and Calvin denounced the retarded as 'filled with satan'" (Rosen et al, 1976, p xiii), which demonisation did not begin to change until the 18th century (Rosen et al, 1976, p xiii).

Wear (1992, p 124) specifies childbirth and death as two important life events that were less medicalised in early modern times than today. Death was "a largely non-medical ceremony in the sixteenth and in the first half of the seventeenth century.... Both religions insisted that a priest or minister should be in charge at the deathbed, the medical practitioner having departed when it was clear that no more could be done medically.... The process of dying was part of social life", with family and friends present, as well as the priest or minister.

Religious emphasis reduced in the latter half of the 17th century and by the latter half of the 18th century a medicalised death was forming. Citing Porter and Porter, Wear (1992, p 125) states that "some doctors remained at the deathbed and 'managed' death, using opiates to deaden pain. But in doing so they reduced both the independence of the dying and their role in the process of dying". The change from religious to medicalised death "reflects and confirms the decline of religion and the process of secularisation which encouraged the medicalisation of life and death" (Wear, 1992, p 125).

This pattern was repeated in care for intellectual disability. In the medieval period, "there is no evidence that they [the 'mentally retarded'] were regarded by physicians as part of their medical responsibility" (Rosen et al, 1976, p xiii). The 18th century saw educational approaches develop. By 1792, the French scientist Pinel "was convinced that the mentally deranged were diseased rather than sinful or immoral" (Rosen et al, 1976, p xiv). The educational approach became emphasised in the mid-19th century throughout the US and Europe with the establishment of special schools that became the (medical or religio-medical) institutions of the 20th century (Ferleger and Boyd, 1980, p 166), as has been mentioned.

The physical reductionism of medicine conceives of disease as residing within the individual, caused and cured within the individual. The social causes of disease and the social definition of disease and the body are almost immaterial. As Zola (1977, p 63) explains, medicine scapegoats the sick, and therefore deviant, individual. If deviant individuals are sick, then social, economic and political systems do not have to examine their involvement in creating these individuals. And as McKnight (1977) says, the 'answer' or 'cure' lies with the professional and no one else. Wolfensberger (1992a, pp 7-8) also notes scapegoating as one of three functional reasons why societies 'need' deviant classes. The moral neutrality of medicine has shifted the notion of morality, positioning medicine as the definer of "what can and should be eliminated" (Zola, 1977, p 63). Medicine is the modern definer of deviance (Zola, 1972; Conrad and Schneider, 1980).

Care of the body, care of the soul

All medieval hospitals aimed to care for the soul as well as the body through a series of religious obligations (Bailey, 1988). The aim to care for body and soul was transferred directly into the later medical hospitals that began around the beginning of the 18th century. In these institutions, as Bailey's (1988, p 162) examples illustrate, the care of the inmates' religion and morals was at least as important as caring for their bodies.

The ancient Christian dichotomy of 'care versus cure' persisted throughout the medieval period. The use of witchcraft and members of the local community to assist in treatment sat alongside the use of authorised and unauthorised medical care (Park, 1992). With medicine itself including magic and religious healing, treating the soul inevitably accompanied treating the body. From the late 14th century, "appeals to supernatural forces gradually became a hallmark of the illegitimate practitioner or charlatan, at least in the eyes of city authorities" (Park, 1992, p 82).

Christianity achieved dominance in Europe in the early Middle Ages. The Christian ministry, "the prototype of all professions", was deeply enmeshed in communal life (Zola, 1977, p 43). Aries (cited in Prior, 1989, p 154) identifies the 13th century as the time when the belief in the separation of the soul from the body at death arose, and as the time when the clericalisation of the funeral took place. Prior (1989, p 167) shows that modern Irish Catholics believe in the ancient idea of a human totality, a body–soul unity before and after death, in contrast to Protestants who conceive the soul as separating from the body at death.

Although the Church did play a key role in the provision of medical and hospital care, the role of the Church in establishing medieval hospitals has been over-emphasised. Hospitals did not grow out of the early Church hospices. Hospitals became prominent because a "leading lay person or group would decide on the need for a hospital" (Granshaw,

1992, p 201). Granshaw (1992, p 200) states: "To their endowers, [medieval and early modern] hospitals were intended more for the cure of souls than of bodies". Porter (1992b, p 108) suggests secularisation could be involved in the 18th-century preoccupation with health and the body.

From the 17th century the body–mind dichotomy at the root of modern science enabled the body and mind to be considered as distinct compartments of the person. The further compartmentalisation of the person due to professionalisation can be seen, according to McKnight (1977), as deriving from specialisation in medicine and the development of the medico-psychological and social welfare professions. In late modernity, the needs of the body and of the soul require an interdisciplinary professional team (Illich, 1977). A team of professionals has replaced the priest or minister. The medico-psychological disciplines somatise the soul. Because the biochemistry of the brain is believed to disclose and operationalise the psyche, the care of the soul now involves another psychophysical set of compartments for a residual group of deviant symptoms or behaviours in the medicalised care of the body.

In relation to the care of the souls of the dead, Aries (1981) charts the changes in the management of the dead in the West. In broad terms, the dead were shifted: from being inside the city walls to being outside them; from being on sanctified ground or inside churches to being outside them and then, later, in segregated cemeteries. Cemeteries themselves shifted from being open and integrated public spaces to being closed and high walled; from being a central focus of religious, civic and social life to serving the specific function of housing the dead. In a study of Belfast, Prior (1989) confirms various aspects of these shifts in the medieval and modern period. Prior (1989) finds one final segregation of the dead that reflects the modern vision, the isolation of the dead from each other in separate, individual graves.

Philanthropic connections

Self-interest

The medieval period is marked by the establishment of hospitals by private benefactors. In the 15th century, hospitals were mainly established either by the bishop of the diocese, the merchant guild or the private benefactor, the Crown also playing some role (Cartwright, 1977, pp 24-5, 30). Abuse of hospitals' finances caused the Crown to assume ownership and change the purpose of many hospitals

(Cartwright, 1977, pp 30-2). Following the Dissolution, whose purpose was to destroy the power of the Catholic Church and increase Protestant and treasury wealth, the dearth of care necessitated a reorganisation. More than a century later all that had occurred was that the few institutions that had survived were renamed (Cartwright, 1977, pp 32-5), "the only certain exception is Bridewell, little better than a whipping-house for beggars and prostitutes" (Cartwright, 1977, p 35).

The philanthropic connection of the hospital system served the interests of benefactors. Benefactors used charitable works to ensure heavenly reward as well as to assure their earthly memory in perpetuity (Bailey, 1988; Granshaw, 1989a). Broadly speaking, it was not the needs of the destitute but self-interest that motivated private benefactors.

In modern times, philanthropy served variously the self-interest of capitalism, industrialisation and aristocratic elites, as well as that of benefactors themselves. In France in the 16th century, many ecclesiastical hospitals were transferred into municipal hands. British prosperity increased dramatically in the early 18th century and travellers to the continent could only be impressed by its hospital systems. As a result, wealthy individuals began to establish the English voluntary hospitals beginning in the 18th century (Cartwright, 1977, p 36). However, "it was to be many years before the hospital developed from a house for lodging the sick into an institution for the cure of disease" (Cartwright, 1977, p 39).

In the mid-18th century medical men colonised infirmaries (Porter, 1989, pp 159-61). Asylums were already under medical control. The 19th century saw medical men become entrepreneurs. Hospitals were founded by medical men for their social and professional advancement (Granshaw, 1992) and continued to be founded by the wealthy. The respectability and high social status attaching to philanthropy assisted the attainment of high social status for the hospital as an institution, as well as for doctors. The state maintained its role under the Poor Laws. Australia did not import the machinery of the Poor Law (Evans, 1983, p 205). The newly acquired penal colony adopted a similar approach to the private charity model of the English system whose central feature was the voluntary hospital (Crichton, 1990, p 11). However, in Australia the reliance on philanthropy by the wealthy, the churches and charitable foundations was emphasised to compensate for the absence of Poor Relief funds from taxation. Because Australia did not have the same option as the English voluntary hospitals of sending unwanted, prospective patients to Poor Law workhouses and their infirmaries, the difficulty of determining who should receive the privilege of care, and so the importance of philanthropic, medical and governmental screening processes, was also emphasised (Crichton, 1990, p 14).

Privilege versus right

The premise behind the establishment of the early hospitals was that people needed to be separated from everyday life to recover, which was by no means the rule since all hospitals had significant death rates. In large part recovery was no doubt due to the improved living conditions in institutional care (Rubin, 1989, p 51). Formal care was a privilege. By the end of the Middle Ages the philanthropic establishment of hospitals had resulted in a few receiving a great deal and many more receiving very little (Bailey, 1988).

Szasz (1994) characterises the modern shift away from medieval philanthropy in the following way. "So long as that [poor relief a religious duty to God rather than to the poor themselves] was the case, the engine of poor relief was driven more by the donors' rectitude than by the recipients' need; and the donors, feeling ennobled by their charitableness, were relatively unconcerned about the corrupting effect of the dole on the pauper's character." However, "helping the poor by giving charity salves the person's conscience. Being taxed so the state can support parasites vexes a person's soul" (Szasz, 1994, p 17).

The key right attending hospital philanthropy was the right to determine who could receive care by, in the first instance, the benefactor determining that a facility of a certain type would be built and, then, by holding the right to nominate and approve inmates. Arguments about the non-deserving poor abusing the provision of care abound under the philanthropic model in the modern period. The screening or selection process remained the key feature of this model. Medical screening then provided a second means to sort out who was entitled to care. Incurables and the chronically and terminally ill were generally excluded from the privilege of care. Grateful servility has always been the response demanded for the gift of care.

THREE

Palliative care

Introduction

Being part of the care system, palliative care expresses and interprets its mission within the paradigm of care. The historical development of palliative care is bounded by this constriction. A paradigmatic analysis of palliative care shows how palliative care gives expression to the constraints of the broader paradigm of care. The practice of contemporary palliative care also exhibits, in general terms, the detrimental effects of the broader paradigm. Problems, therefore, arise from palliative care's conformity to the paradigm of care.

This chapter aims to develop a brief paradigmatic analysis of palliative care using the same framework that was derived for care in general, in Chapter Two (refer 'Paradigmatic analysis' section). In addition, this chapter aims to identify the key problems arising from the transference into palliative care of the detrimental effects of the paradigm of care.

It is argued that the paradigm of palliative care strongly exhibits all the major features of the broader paradigm of care. The main detrimental effect of the paradigm of care is to establish and validate the distinction between a socially valued class of care providers such as doctors or philanthropists and a socially devalued class of care recipients and people excluded from care. As the social organisation of care becomes more modern and industrialised, this distinction becomes increasingly pronounced. Wide-ranging institutionalisation of devalued people becomes the preferred form of social management in modern times. The social devaluation of people who receive care becomes more pronounced and systematised with the increasing dominance of the institutional model of care.

This central defect is also pronounced in palliative care, through its conformity with the broader paradigm. The social devaluation of people who are dying is perpetuated by the way modern palliative care is originally conceived and by the way it continues to be constructed. The key problem, therefore, is that there is a fundamental contradiction between palliative care ideals and its definition, organisation and practice.

This chapter is divided into two sections. The first section, 'Paradigm of palliative care', develops a brief paradigmatic analysis of palliative care, using the same key features and sub-headings as for the paradigm of care in the previous chapter (refer 'Paradigmatic analysis' section). The second section, 'Problem for palliative care', examines the problematic implications of the palliative care paradigm using the same scheme.

Paradigm of palliative care

At the beginning of each of the following theme sub-headings, such as 'Religion and medicine', for each key feature a one-paragraph summary is given of the key developments in the paradigm of care from Chapter Two. These brief summaries serve to recap major trends from Chapter Two to assist in understanding how palliative care reflects these broad trends in the area described in each sub-heading.

Institutional expression and role system

Religion and medicine

Institutional expression in care shifts from a religious context to a medical one. Much of the institutional function of religion is assumed by medicine and a medicalised, and medico-psychologised, context of care and life in modernity. The moral neutrality of medicine allows moral concerns in regard to care, particularly those of religion, to be bracketed out of consideration.

Palliative care through its medical and medico-psychological aspects absorbs and expresses the quasi-religious implications of medicine. Seale (1998) describes the prescriptions of the new psychologism of the late modern period with respect to palliative care. Dying and death, which are central to all religion and especially central to Christianity (Kaufmann, 1976, pp xix, 224), are now medical and medico-psychological problems, as well as religious ones. There are now medical options to transcend death (Kearl, 1989, p 412) and it is now the doctor who is engaged in the battle against death (Kearl, 1989, p 423).

The hospital and nursing home replace the monastic and lay infirmary, the medieval hospice and almshouse. In palliative care, the modern hospice substitutes for the hospital, at least initially and symbolically. Palliative care creates its own therapeutic institution and institutes its own kind of therapeutic community with religious and philanthropic overtones. A segregated religio-therapeutic community is premised on the belief that inmates need to be separated from their everyday life in their normal community to be made whole by a specialised group who know how to care for body and soul. This premise requires that the everyday relationships and interactions between people receiving care and their normal community, which can only occur within that community, are replaced to some degree, usually considerably, by 'special', newly found and often paid-for interactions in an artificial, segregated community of carers.

Authority, status and respectability

Institutional expression in care is associated with conferring authority, status, respectability and social approval on the pattern of care incorporated in the institution, and also on the institution itself. Since a pattern of adopting certain social forms necessarily involves the exclusion of alternative forms with opposite features, informal and non-institutional patterns of care are, therefore, conferred a lower authority, status, respectability and social approval. The lay health culture of informal care, multiple practitioners with overlapping roles and self-medication remains a constant counterposed feature to the ever more differentiated patterns of formal care. In modernity, with the increasing monopoly of the medical industry by the medical profession, lay health culture becomes increasingly socially devalued, akin to quackery or, at least, amateurism. Institutional expression facilitates market expansionism and monopolisation as evidenced, for example, in the expansion of psychiatric territory throughout the 20th century, the victory of the medicalised model of 'madness' in the 19th century and the victory of the general over the specialist hospital in the 19th and 20th centuries. Institutional care is seen as the best means to provide care. Aspects of care that cannot profit institutional agenda are not provided by the institution, such as care for 'incurables' once cure, in the form of acute care, becomes dominant. 'Incurables' in late modernity exist as such only 'provisionally' because medicalisation implies illness, treatment and cure.

By the early 20th century there are several homes for people who are dying. The Sisters of Charity resurrect the word 'hospice' to name its homes for the dying of the late 19th and early 20th centuries in Ireland and England (Saunders, 1977). "Research into the control of terminal cancer pain began at St Luke's Hospital in 1948, and was developed at St Joseph's Hospice between 1958 and 1965 by Cicely (now Dame) Saunders" (Murphy, 1989, p 235). In 1967,

St Christopher's Hospice is established "as the first research and teaching hospice" (Murphy, 1989, p 236).

Clark (1993, p 169) asserts "the need to more actively promote strategies for community care of dying people [due to] some new hospices [having a] vision of, and system of care more appropriate to, the understanding of 1970s than the 1990s". The marginalisation of community palliative care seems to continue. Commenting that in his survey of 43 new hospices nearly 80% were seeking to provide inpatient services and 90% day care, Clark (1993, p 169) notes that the desire to provide day care has caused little "diminution" of the desire to build inpatient services. He states: "although hospice is often described as a 'philosophy and not a place', the continuing emphasis on traditional forms of inpatient care and on the 'bricks and mortar' of provision is striking" (Clark, 1993, p 169). Clark and Seymour's (1999, p 151) later conclusion, based on more extensive UK data from 1965-98, is that "all forms of palliative care delivery have grown rapidly since 1965, but that home support has grown most significantly". However, the data do not appear to support this conclusion, except in the most rudimentary manner that home support services are the most numerous in 1998. Although there is dubious statistical validity in measuring the comparative growth rates of hospice service types by using the sheer number of each service type, as Clark and Seymour (1999, pp 74, 151) appear to do, the author's approximate statistical analysis of Clark and Seymour's (1999, p 74) data on that basis shows no time period where home support has grown more significantly than all other service types, except for periods prior to 1985 in which trends involve massive and atypical growth rates due to the numbers being so small.

Again, although statistically problematic in terms of validity, using the number of each service type to calculate comparative growth rates for US data from the Hospice Association of America (2002) for 1986-2001 paints what may be a more likely overall picture. For 1990-2001, Medicare-certified hospice service types' comparative growth rates are: 67% (skilled nursing facility-based), 121% (home health agency-based), 150% (hospital based) and 286% (freestanding hospices). In the latter half of this period, 1996-2001, both the growth of hospital-based and skilled nursing facility-based services appears to be ceasing, if not declining. However, the number of freestanding hospices *increases* by 26.8%, while the number of home health agency-based hospice services *decreases* by 15.3% to 1994-95 levels. Freestanding hospices are also the only service type that has grown every year from 1986 to 2001.

Although the proliferation and intransigence of the institutional model in palliative care are striking, they are by no means surprising since they are highly effective means for achieving institutional ends. For palliative care, seeking credibility, authority and status including recognition within the medical mainstream, the institutional model is the established means to achieve these ends.

The philanthropic connections and religious connotations of the voluntary and specialist hospital systems, in particular, have been used to forge a path to authority, status and respectability for palliative care. The saints' names of many of the voluntary and specialist hospitals, and now hospices, allude to this fact. The 'bricks and mortar' method noted by Clark (1993, p 169) is the well-trodden path. This 1860 *British Medical Journal* term (Granshaw, 1989b, p 216) is also used by Granshaw (1989b) to describe the way specialist hospitals and doctors in the 19th century achieved authority and respectability. This same path to the same ends is being forged by palliative care, which has added to this well-trodden path the recent tool of a multidisciplinary team based on the scientific, medical approach.

Social responsibility and social control

Institutional expression facilitates specialisation and professionalisation and other outcomes, such as philanthropic sponsorship, which promotes social acceptance and credibility. In short, institutional expression in care conveys the message that the particular social problem should be solved, indeed can be and is being solved, by the means instituted. The extent to which institutional expression in an area of care is religious and, in modernity, medical and medico-psychological, indicates the propensity for that area of care to designate what is a social problem and what is not. Such institutional expression becomes socially authorised to handle and regulate the problem or deviance, and is expected to do so.

The idea of social responsibility contains the idea of social control. An institution assumes the social responsibility to manage a condition that causes social concern, such as poverty or illness. If it does not exercise proper social control, the institution acts irresponsibly. 'Medicine as an institution of social control' is viewed negatively by Zola (1972) because, while medicine has a proper responsibility to control the conditions surrounding illness, the definition of illness has been expanded inappropriately to cover every facet of living, at least potentially. Excessive social control signifies that other factors, such as institutional agenda, are taking precedence over social responsibility.

Palliative care has gained almost universal social approval (Doyle,

1999). Its social responsibility is highly valued. At the same time palliative care acts inevitably as a means to regulate the condition of dying. As a late modern form, with significant institutional, medical and professional expression, it must serve social control functions and reflect the moral dilemmas surrounding "medicine as an institution of social control", to use Zola's (1972) phrase. For late modernity, control over future events is a central concern (Seale, 1998, p 84). Palliative care is used to control the future in the sphere of dying, in the sense that the process of dying is standardised and socially managed by palliative care. Palliative care assists to control the social disturbances caused by death and dying and enables social disquiet arising from attendant conditions, such as bereavement, to dissipate. Referring to Turner (1969), Prior (1989, p 157) indicates that death, as a liminal state, is perceived as dangerous since it opposes structure and permanence. Importantly, palliative care may be used to control this danger of liminality by conforming the social understanding and manifestation of death and dying. Referring to original work by Froggatt (1997) and Lawton (1998), Seale (1998, p 119) suggests "hospice care ... might be usefully understood as an institutional construction of liminal space". Palliative care, by definition, manages death and dying in socially valued ways and excludes management of death and dying in socially devalued ways. Kellehear (1990, p 194) has noted aspects of this social pressure on people who are dying to achieve the socially defined 'good death', but not with respect to the pressure from palliative care itself. Lofland (1978) analyses the cultural or ideological prescriptions of the 'happy death movement', to use her words. Seale (1998) continues this type of analysis concerned with the scripts or roles prescribed by palliative care. These prescriptions allow what palliative care values, and disallow what it does not value. Clark and Seymour (1999) provide further commentary about palliative care prescriptions concerning the 'good death'.

Role system and obligations

Institutions of care are modelled on religious institutions, including their religious ethos and the idea of a religious community. Institutional role systems involve a hierarchical ordering of a 'therapeutic' community with a strong emphasis on vocational and religious mission. Institutional roles are strictly defined. The inmate role is especially strictly defined and centres on the obligation to comply and express gratitude. Particularly since medicine has quasi-religious significance in modern times, the shift in power in doctor–patient relationships around the early 19th century intensifies the pre-existing obligations of gratitude and compliance. Inmate role conformity in institutional care is very strict, and has been so for a very long time.

Patient role definition in hospitals is an important element in understanding the workings of the modern hospital including the interpersonal interactions among staff and patients. The question as to what role definition is imposed by the hospice as institution or specialist hospital, and hospice care as a mode of care, has been examined to some degree by Lofland (1978), Backer et al (1982, p 55) and Seale (1998). Glaser and Strauss (1965, 1968), Charmaz (1980) and Field (1989) are among others for whom the complex interplay of role system and power in interpersonal interaction holds a central place.

In palliative care, the funds derived from voluntary donations, especially from deceased estates, are an obvious starting point for examining issues concerning obligation and gratitude. The historical significance of the deceased estate to ensure the material well-being of survivors and the spiritual well-being of the deceased (Aries, 1981), the former purpose (at least) still routinely persisting (Kellehear, 1990), raises questions about the appropriateness of palliative care benefiting from donations from the deceased estate or the bereaved. To the extent that palliative care is perceived as a gift, there is implicit inducement to donate to repay that gift. Palliative care's pronounced voluntary staff component supports the perception of palliative care as a gift, as do contributions from philanthropic sources. St Christopher's Hospice, the international hospice care emblem and model, raises funds from both second-hand shops and corporate support (St Christopher's Hospice, 2003a). The hospice also fund-raises using collection boxes, the archetypal religious and charitable way of donation, as well as suggesting people remember St Christopher's in their wills (St Christopher's Hospice, 2003a).

St Christopher's Hospice is explicitly and fundamentally a "Christian and medical foundation", as Saunders states (cited in Bradshaw, 1996, p 412). The sense of vocation and religious mission is naturally also pronounced (Saunders, 1977; Bradshaw, 1996). As such, St Christopher's reproduction throughout hospice culture generally incorporates both religion and medicine into the basis of hospice. The influence of these key elements of the paradigm of care, therefore, pervades palliative care, the prescription of rigid roles, strict compliance and gratitude for care being illustrations. The critical feature incorporated into the very basis of palliative care by this pairing of religion and medicine under an institutional management model is the social devaluation of people receiving care that attends these models in modernity in particular.

Prescriptive roles arise in relation to many contexts in palliative care. The typical US hospice patient is white with cancer, "the percentage of women being slightly greater than that of men" (Mor and Masterson–Allen, 1987, p 39). Cultural exclusivity problems (for example Hill and Penso, 1995, cited in Bosanquet and Salisbury, 1999, p 35; Gordon, 1996, cited in Robbins, 1998, p 119; Smaje and Field, 1997; Prior, 1999a, 1999b) raise questions about role stereotyping, prescribed behaviours and the ways in which marginalisation is operationalised in palliative care. Institutional expression raises questions about role conformity, compliance and gratitude, and questions about the prescribed notions concerning non–institutional care.

Religious ethos

Gift of charity

Christianity in the West is intimately connected with care. The authority, power and respectability of religion are attached to the institutions of care. The hospital and its community are modelled on religious organisations and communities. A religious ethos accompanies the idea of care, as does the sense of vocation and religious mission. The religious ethos involves charity and an inversion of values where the recipient of care is idealised as an opportunity for religiously inspired action on the part of the carer, or as the bearer of a special wisdom able to teach some sort of lesson.

To repeat, St Christopher's Hospice is a "Christian and medical foundation" (Saunders, 1986, p 42, cited in Bradshaw, 1996, p 412), and each of its five fundamental principles expresses the elements of the religious ethos in palliative care (Saunders, 1986, p 45, cited in Bradshaw, 1996, p 412), which Bradshaw characterises as "love in action" (Bradshaw, 1996, p 412). The romantic idealisation of recipients of care in palliative care is evident, for example, in its portrayal of the "dying hero" (Seale, 1998, p 92), in the numerous personal accounts and anecdotes in the literature (for example, in Saunders, 1977; Moller, 1996) and in the perception that palliative care clients, staff and services are 'special', for example, 'Very Special Kids' (Very Special Kids, 2003). People with an intellectual disability are also euphemistically called 'very special' people, or people with 'special' needs. Lofland (1978) was one of the first to understand that the almost obligatory paradoxical titles of much of the death and dying literature convey a mystification and idealisation of death and dying, and of palliative care, via the implication that palliative care possesses a knowledge that involves a reversal of conventional wisdom and a resolution of opposites. *Dying they live: St Christopher's Hospice* (Saunders, 1977) and *Death: The final stage of growth* (Kubler-Ross, 1975) are prominent examples.

The sense of mission in palliative care is a renewal of the religious calling so intimately involved with care and exhibited strongly in the case of Nightingale and the hospital/nursing orders. Originally in palliative care, those with a vocation were sought more than those with qualifications (Rumbold, 1999). A therapeutic community could then be built based on a calling from God, as in medieval times, rather than on secular criteria divorced from the sense of religious mission.

Morality and meaning

The religious context of death and dying shifts to a medicalised one. As disease is believed to reside within the individual in modernity, so too the soul or mind is believed to reside within the individual, usually within the brain. The meaning of morality and disease becomes clouded by the medical and medico-psychological context because its determinations are portrayed as scientific and objective and, therefore, morally neutral.

The idea that disease is an abnormality within a part of the physical body is central to modern medical science (Prior, 1989, p 200). According to Prior (1989, p 132), "death in the modern world is seen basically as an abnormality, not just a product of disease but a disease itself [and] after all, death only finds itself in hospital because we have a vision of it as an untimely event brought on by disease". Prior (1989, p 130) finds it both "strange and significant" that the hospice movement should hide death in a segregated therapeutic space akin to the hospital it sought to reform. He goes on to assert that dying, unlike other illness groups, has not been segregated in a hospital department because a specific therapy for dying has not existed. According to Prior, dying is segregated in hospitals "in a much finer mesh" (Prior, 1989, p 130), such as the dying room. Now that hospice care has found a 'dying therapy', the hospital can segregate people who are dying within its walls via inpatient palliative care units. Not only is the hospital monopoly secured thereby but more importantly, segregation of dying can become universally applied, as does the institutional identification of dying with abnormality and the triad sickness, therapy or treatment, and cure. Such 'universal access' to palliative care means universal segregation and devaluation via the sick role alone, if via no other.

The idea of progress and attainment as the result of effort is central to modernist thought. In discussing the influence of the Protestant work ethic on understanding grief, Charmaz (1980) notes that grief is now inside us, like disease. Prior (1989) is one of many authors who concur. The socially valued modern response to grief is the medico-psychological one known as 'grief work'. This work corresponds in some ways to the inner spiritual work of Christianity. However, while the medico-psychological approaches "offer the self as an object of worship" as Seale (1998, p 62) remarks, traditional inner Christian work offers Christ as that object. Palliative care exemplifies the confluence of medico-psychological approaches with some aspects of traditional religious approaches, including the belief in the moral virtue of emotional or psychological work, which both approaches involve. The late modern discourses concerning grief make it very clear that grief is now constructed as "hard work" (Seale, 1998, pp 106, 197).

The profound meaning, value and place of suffering are essential to Christianity and to care. The meaning of death and dying is inextricably interwoven in Christianity with the death and sacrifice of Christ and the value of His suffering and death as the redemptive act. Medicine, including the medico-psychological disciplines, has anaesthetised, sanitised and standardised suffering, termed the 'killing of pain' by Illich (1976). The moral neutrality of medicine sees pain and suffering as aberrant symptoms to be cured, palliated or even anaesthetised. In the process Christian moral perspectives, which centre on the value and meaning for our lives of Christ's suffering and, thus, that of our own and others' suffering, become side issues.

Care of the body, care of the soul

Integrated ways of caring for body and soul become at least theoretically differentiated under the Christian influence where care is directed more toward the good of the soul than toward bodily cure. In modernity, the body–mind dichotomy underlying scientific thought allows the identification of the mind with the brain and, therefore, the soul with the rational mind. The soul is reduced to a somatic principle under the medico-psychological approaches. The age-old idea of care for a unified body–soul becomes a compartmentalised care for the body combined with a compartmentalised care for the rationality of mind. The specialisation of medicine compartmentalises the body and the rationality of mind. Medicine assumes all care for the body and soul. Care reduces to cure, with acute approaches dominating the landscape of care.

Palliative care, through its medical and medico-psychological expression and through its incorporation of a team of professionals, implies that the aspects of the process of dying can be compartmentalised into a discrete set of problems, issues or symptoms. The stage theories of grief and loss are the most obvious examples that try to squeeze human experience into a set of theoretical compartments. As another related example, Moller (1996, p 131) regrets that "by turning the experience of grief and bereavement into distinct and compartmentalised research questions, thanatologists tend to trivialise the human experience of grief". The idea of 'total pain' (Saunders and Baines, 1983, pp 14, 43-50), the expectation of blurred team member roles and the team meeting process in palliative care attest to the need to try to reintegrate what the concepts, structures and processes of palliative care tend to separate and compartmentalise.

Concerning the modern compartmentalisation of the dead, the social organisation of this aspect of care shifts from the dead being integrated physically, socially and spiritually within the community of the living to a physically, socially and spiritually segregated community in cemeteries outside towns. This shift from community integration to marginalisation demonstrates a shift toward the social devaluation of the community of the dead. Prior (1989, p 157) emphasises this shift, in explaining that high status individuals rarely come into physical contact with the dead, stating that "it is death as a social category rather than as a physical phenomenon that is truly the pollutant". Having recently displaced earlier informal patterns, such as those of kinship groups (Prior 1989) or the neighbourhood layer-out (Addams, 1993), the funeral industry assists in the fragmentation of the process of dying and death.

Philanthropic connections

Self-interest

The contribution of philanthropy to the development of care is a dominant feature of the paradigm of care. In addition, a dominant feature of this involvement is that philanthropists' interests are served by their efforts rather than the interest of the recipients of care. Seeking more balance in the widespread assessment of philanthropists as self-serving, Bailey (1988) stresses that, broadly speaking, humanitarian sentiments are also involved. Nevertheless philanthropists' personal gain is generally very significant and can only be fully judged in terms of the value each individual places on the heavenly insurance believed to be won by charitable works. The social outcomes of charitable efforts on the other hand, such as doctors acquiring gentlemanly status or capitalists ensuring a sufficient labour force, are indisputably in philanthropists' own interests.

Philanthropic self-interest does not seem especially marked in the development of palliative care in general. However, the level of philanthropic involvement in palliative care is especially marked. In examining the research evidence, Robbins (1998, pp 123-4) indicates that, for Britain, "because hospices receive a substantial amount of their revenue (on average about 50 per cent) from charitable sources [charitable foundations, fundraising, donations and legacies], as well as accruing cost savings through the use of volunteer labour, they provide a subsidised service to health district residents in terms of costs borne by the statutory sector". The purpose of philanthropy needs to be understood within the broader context of self-interest, such as the convergence of the interests of palliative care services and the state in this case. Voluntary contributions, such as volunteer labour, also need to be understood within the obligation of gratitude to palliative care providers.

With the extensive involvement of the state in managing care, the eminence of the social status attaching to the philanthropist has been moderated. In late modernity, eminent social status for philanthropists attaches to only the most socially approved causes, such as palliative care, in contrast to aged care, psychiatric care or intellectual disability services, for example. This elevation of palliative care derives from it combining the twin 'religious' elements of religion and modern medicine. The ennoblement of palliative care arises from romantic idealisations associated with both its religious and its medical and medico-psychological elements, as well as from the institutional authority attending them. Now that cancer has become curable by modern medicine to some degree, the great fear and stigma surrounding cancer mean that those who fight against cancer or those who care for people with cancer are idealised, including those involved philanthropically. Palliative care is one such field idealised and ennobled by its focus on cancer and its search for a way to make dying of cancer more palatable.

Privilege versus right

The chief right attaching to philanthropy is the right to determine which groups and individuals are able to receive care. One key purpose of benefaction is to screen selection, to separate the deserving from the undeserving. The connection between philanthropy and care cements the idea of care as a privilege bestowed by those who can and should provide care. With this inherited bias, asserting care as a right is problematic. Philanthropic, charitable or voluntary connotations evoke the 'gift relation' (Porter, 1989). The strict obligations to compliance, servility and gratitude of the inmate role are intimately bound up with the privilege of care.

The connection via philanthropy between care and religious, aristocratic, social and economic elites, and also, in later times, between care and medical and bureaucratic elites, confers institutional authority, power, status and respectability to the institutions of care and their way of managing and delivering care. With such an interrelationship, a central characteristic of care involves the juxtaposition of the powerful and the powerless, a socially valued donor (or provider) class and a socially devalued beneficiary (or recipient) class and an underclass of devalued groups excluded from care altogether. Through its religious ethos and strong religio-charitable connotations, palliative care implies this characteristic of the charitable model of the revered givers and the pitiful burdens of charity.

With the state taking over the funding of hospitals and palliative care services, the state, as philanthropist, retains the bureaucratic privilege to determine client selection criteria, to set limits to the amount and type of care provided and to assess quality of care. The modern state is not disinterested, but seeks, if nothing else, to rationalise healthcare budgets. State funding from general revenue markedly standardises the philanthropic connection and removes some of the stigma from burdens of charity. Nevertheless, the economic interests of the state and the professional service industry are well served by the provision of care, as McKnight (1977) asserts. In addition, Navarro (1976) demonstrates that in the US the elite classes are deeply entrenched in the medical industry and in government. He indicates that, as a result, the elite classes' economic and political interests are also well served by the modern healthcare industry. As palliative care becomes more a part of the healthcare mainstream, these broad issues can have an increasing impact.

Problem for palliative care

Institutional expression and role system

Religion and medicine

Until recently, religion has always been the definer of human identity. The value or goodness attaching to professionals, and human service organisations, is at the root of the problem of understanding what is occurring in medicine and care in modernity and what is at stake, as Zola (1972) realises. The medical arena is the example par excellence of the modern battle for control of the definition of human identity "not because the perspective, tools and practitioners of medicine and the other helping professions are evil, but because they are not" (Zola, 1972, p 502). The ideological prescription of identity by medical and medico-psychological discourse is almost invisible. The danger that the 'banality of evil' (Arendt, 1963, cited in Zola, 1972, p 502) will become entrenched in medical and medico-psychological care is great because "not only is the process masked as a technical, scientific, objective one, but one done for our own good" (Zola, 1972, p 502).

The same applies to palliative care in so far as it involves medical and medico-psychological expression. Much more dangerous than the complacency mentioned by Doyle (1990) is the 'odour of goodness' that pervades the hospice movement and upsets many of its members, according to Smith (1984). Douglas (1992, p 579) describes hospice care as "too good to be true". Clark's (1993, pp 173-4) discussion states Douglas' crucial question: "why should collective dying be a good thing?".

After reporting various responses to Douglas (1992) with some bearing on Douglas' criticism, Clark then points to "Douglas's well-known and widespread error of equating hospice with a building, rather than a programme of cure [sic] ... deliverable in a wide range of settings" (Clark 1993, p 173) (although Clark obviously means 'care' not 'cure'). Clark invokes this palliative care dogma, often repeated by Saunders (Bradshaw, 1996, p 412), which divorces programmes from their contexts. Douglas' key assertion, that hospices as specialist institutions for group dying are neither necessary nor desirable, can thus be portrayed as empty or plainly misinformed.

However, Douglas does not in any way fail to understand that hospice is a programme of care able to be applied in various settings. On the contrary, he explicitly describes quite valid components of a palliative care programme that he would value. Moreover, he explains that he would only value such a programme if it were delivered from a general hospital via the medical mainstream rather than from a hospice. Douglas' view reflects a general one within the medical mainstream, as Clark (1993, p 173) notes, and as such echoes the battle won by the medical establishment and general hospital over the specialist hospital in the 19th and 20th centuries. The greatest significance of Douglas' (1992) comments is that he disputes the core hospice wisdom that group dying is good and that hospices are necessary.

The goodness of palliative care and its religious ethos mean criticism can be too easily dismissed as misinformed, missing the point or merely argumentative. Dismissing the criticism of medicalisation by Biswas (1993), a nurse, Ahmedzai (1993) tends to invoke the authority and prestige of the doctor to try to reassure that medicalisation of palliative care, if it exists at all, is absolutely nothing to worry about. Ahmedzai sees goodness in medicalisation and in palliative care. To others like Biswas (1993) or Bradshaw (1996), the goodness attaching to medicalisation, professionalisation or bureaucratisation is bad, relative to the goodness of the true hospice ethos. Clark and Seymour's (1999) examination of the medicalisation and "routinisation" (James and Field, 1992) theses demonstrates definitional and other confusions in palliative care regarding these issues. More generally, Clark and Seymour (1999, p 180) find that "the practice of palliative care is surrounded by some important definitional and etymological problems".

The perception of the goodness of medicalisation raises complex social issues. In the past, religion determined good and bad, normal and deviant. Medicine has taken over this role to a substantial degree in late modernity. Because irrationality is the key descriptor of deviance in modernity (Porter, 1992a), its deviance as 'insanity' has been medicalised via the medico-psychological disciplines. Similarly, the irrationality of death, its inexplicability, insolubility and unpredictability, signifies to modernity the deviance of death and dying. Wolfensberger suggests the reason there are dying rooms in hospitals is to segregate the person who is dying so as to "save us the unpleasantness of ultimate deviancy" (Wolfensberger, 1972, p 24). The deviance of death and dying creates a significant impetus toward medicalisation and, in general, a rationalisation of death and dying through formal social management.

The marriage in palliative care of the religious imprimatur with the modern medical and quasi-religious imprimatur sends a powerful symbolic message that the hospice possesses the solutions to dying and death and can control their deviance. By intermingling religion with medicine, modern palliative care obfuscates the social, moral and spiritual meaning of death. The physical reductionism of medicine tends to reduce this meaning to the individual level and to the clinical control of a set of holistic symptoms.

The supposed moral neutrality of medical determinations in modernity raises a critical dilemma confronting any reform movement, such as palliative care, that seeks to make medical care more responsive to moral aspects of care, such as the protection of dignity or the sanctity of life. The history of the management of insanity contains a good example of this dilemma and its repercussions. Reformers outside medicine advocated 'moral therapy' (Porter, 1992a, p 300), such as that of the York Retreat in England at the turn of the 19th century, to try to find alternatives to the horrific abuses in asylums, which were under medical control. Although, as Church (1987, p 113) indicates, moral therapy presumed a moral deficiency, moral therapy shares considerable similarities with palliative care: "an avoidance of force and restraint and the systematic deployment of kindness, reason and humanity, all within a family atmosphere" (Porter, 1992a, p 286). Church (1987, p 113) states that for moral therapy "controlling the social, psychological and physical components of the patient and the environment" lead to rehabilitation. Despite the "thorn in the flesh" that the "high repute and excellent results" of the York Retreat represented to the medicalisation of madness (Porter, 1992a, p 286), all asylums eventually became medical institutions. The management of 'the insane' became increasingly medicalised and so institutionalised within hospitals for 'the insane'. This eventuated despite a radical element within the medical profession that had always claimed asylums must necessarily be "manufactories of madness" because, as Porter's (1992a) reference from 1789 asserts, "mad people herded together would inevitably reduce each other to the lowest common denominator" (Porter, 1992a, p 298). Notwithstanding that in these doctors' minds 'the insane' needed the "moral stimulus of the sane not the inevitable stigma of seclusion", the institutionalisation of 'the insane' in medical institutions was victorious (Porter, 1992a, p 298).

These very arguments have had to be reasserted from the 1960s and are still having to be reasserted, for example by Wolfensberger (1972; 1998, p 120), to try to awaken an awareness of the intrinsic effects of institutional models of care. The medicalised model wins the day without needing to reform because its approaches are assumed moral and good. The example of moral therapy also illustrates the absorption of alternative models of management by institutional models of care.

Authority, status and respectability

The hospice takes patients away from general hospitals, which interferes with their right to the most difficult cases for research and also with the hospital's monopoly of the market. Such action, as well as the development of specialist knowledge, threatens the hospital as the symbol of ultimate medical expertise. Palliative care, as a specialist hospital system with an outpatient and community care component, has colonised a specialised market. These same factors contributed to the absorption of specialist hospitals by the general hospital system to cement the medical elite's institutional monopoly of care.

Modern institutions of care collect people of a certain type together and segregate them. By this means, experimentation and teaching can take place, specialised expertise can be developed, authority, status and respectability can be won, and the particular social problem can be shown to be being controlled in a very public and convincing manner. Placing people who are dying in hospices fits this pattern. Saunders et al (1981, cited in Biswas, 1993, p 136), indicate that a breakaway institution from the NHS, or, that is, the general hospital system, had to be formed so that a proven scientific practice and philosophy for managing death and dying could one day move back into the mainstream. This return of the philosophy, attitudes and approaches of palliative care to hospital care of people who are dying is usually understood to mean doing so while retaining the specialist hospice system.

However, now that palliative care's social approval, credibility and expertise has been established, and now that a significant palliative care market has been established, medicine's institutional model is likely to seek to reabsorb the palliative care emblem and its market, which the general hospital monopoly has to some degree lost. The hospital is likely to seek to colonise only those areas or types of palliative care most profitable to the hospital, financially and institutionally.

Institutional colonisation does not just occur one way, since there are incentives on both sides toward greater institutional power and status. When devalued GPs after status and authority sought incorporation into the medical elite, community medical care gradually became absorbed by the medical model centred on the hospital. Relatively devalued palliative care doctors after status and authority, for themselves and palliative care, are re-enacting this process. However, such a route necessarily imposes significant exclusions onto the conceptualisation and organisation of community medicine and community care for people who are dying. By seeking incorporation into the medical elite, through recognition by the medical establishment of palliative medicine as a specialty, doctors in palliative care are following a well-worn path. This is not to say at all that such doctors are motivated by self-interest but rather to say that the interests of palliative care, conceived as an institutional model of care, are best served by medical recognition. The income and market, and prestige and status of individual doctors and palliative care practitioners generally, is also best served by this means, provided these practitioners work in hospitals or other medically approved institutions.

Patterns such as these do not imply a 'cabal' of doctors plotting to gain status but rather that a successful development is the result of myriad political and individual victories, as de Swaan (1990, p 13) indicates, over alternative ways of development. Because of the history of community-based palliative care provision by GPs, Ahmedzai (1993, p 143) finds it strange first, that the establishment of the specialty of palliative medicine in Britain should come from the Royal College of Physicians rather than from the Royal College of General Practitioners and second, that the accreditation is biased towards hospital doctors and some specialties. Far from being unexpected, these circumstances plainly signify the reassertion of the ascendancy of the authority and status of the medical elite and the institutional medical model centred on the hospital.

The home, community care and outpatient care are virtually impotent in promoting authority, respectability and status for palliative care as a religio-therapeutic, medical community and organisation. A segregated environment specialised in dying not only enables hospice care to be insulated from unwanted aspects of hospital care, it also enables hospice care to become respected and authorised both socially and clinically. Philanthropic connections and religious connotations assist in forging palliative care's path to social acceptance and credibility. For example, Paradis and Cummings (1986) report considerable philanthropic support in establishing the US hospice system, as well as modelling on the religio-medical institution of St Christopher's Hospice. In the US in the 1980s, Gibson (1984a, p 159) indicates that "the hospice movement is creating a death facilitating apparatus which possesses a national organisation and this movement has the support of private foundations, insurance companies, private health industries and the federal government". Having sounded the warning that hospice care has the "financial and institutional potential to bring into being a national euthanasia program" (Gibson 1984a, p 159), Gibson (1984b, p 169) stresses that the economic motive in hospice care, that cost-effectiveness is an inducement to facilitate death, will not go away by returning to non-government-funded hospice services because institutional support for hospice from such sources as insurance companies also views it as a means to reduce medical expenditure.

Commenting that situating hospice beds in specialist palliative care units in hospitals can be seen as making palliative care available to all, Rumbold (1999, p 64) states this shift can also be seen as "the institutional recapture of yet another radical movement". This process can also be conceived as the economic and institutional absorption by medicine of a market competitor. With a more humane approach to dying than acute care, palliative care's absorption signifies the replication of the related trend for the takeover, via medicalisation, of reform that centres on moral issues. Community care's unsuitability to institutional purposes means that the community-focused arms of palliative care are unprofitable in every sense for the hospital. The hospital has to provide only an institutionally useful form of palliative care, that is, clinical, inpatient terminal care, just as the hospice has to do. By this means, the hospital can emasculate the economic threat of the palliative care system vis-à-vis the hospital. The devalued community side of palliative care can then be marginalised from the hospital medical model. Authority, status and respectability will then be transferred to those palliative care units or teams in hospitals, irrespective of where else palliative care is provided, since they will have already captured the institutional emblem of palliative care.

Social responsibility and social control

Palliative care inherits social control functions from medicine since palliative care utilises significant medical personnel and structures. Palliative care, as a medical and medico-psychological specialty, necessarily defines what is normal and abnormal in dying. The medical goal is the proper control of abnormal or deviant symptoms. The treatment of terminal restlessness illustrates how far this determination of what is abnormal can go. Although terminal restlessness is considered a common symptom of dying that does not distress the person who is dying, this symptom is often controlled with drugs because it can be distressing to onlookers. The medical goal is to take away the symptom's aberrant nature. In this example, the aberrant nature of dying is excluded altogether and in principle, the patient being treated, even when there is no clinical need, in order to save others from being disturbed by this sign of dying.

Palliative care represents a clear opportunity for the social control of devalued classes through euthanasia and forms of hastening death. Based on the sanctity of life in Christianity, palliative care's moral abhorrence of euthanasia is compromised by adopting mechanistic measures of the value of a life. Referring to quality of life, Robbins (1998, p 36) states "its definition is notoriously problematic". The tendency toward superficiality in measurement of quality of life in palliative care has been criticised by Tigges (1993, cited in Robbins, 1998, p 55). However, the problem with the idea of quality of life runs far deeper than its superficiality or untrustworthy meaning. Quality of life is a term that dehumanises vulnerable people and affirms the abnormality of their lives by measuring it. Wolfensberger advises: "Let's hang up 'quality of life' as a hopeless term" (Race, 2003, p 197). Wolfensberger shows how 'quality of life' is actually a term that quantifies the value of a life and, therefore, is also a concept that opposes the intrinsic value of a life or the sanctity of life. The value of one life can be compared to that of another, or to some sort of acceptable, that is, socially valued norm of quality of life. And those with more quality of life will be the ones determining the value of those with less quality of life. The less the quality of life, the greater the risk of devaluation.

Through its mechanistic, medical and clinical expression, palliative care embraces quality of life as an idea and weakens or abuses its commitment to the sanctity of life, especially vis-à-vis euthanasia. Wolfensberger (1992a) already finds the socially authorised elimination of devalued people being instituted via socially approved machinery. Fears of palliative care being used in this way, such as those of Gibson (1984a), have significant precedents. To the extent that public health approaches focus on quality of life, these approaches also tend to collude with social forces inimical to difference. More importantly, to the extent that these approaches artificially overlay or impose the social values of the day onto social processes, these approaches mask devaluation in goodness or overall social benefit. Past and present connections between public health and eugenics (such as Pernick, 1997, 2002, 2003; Lippman, 2003), together with the fact that eugenics beliefs are still very much alive (Race, 2004, citing his work in press), caution against ideas that assert an overarching social benefit to all people or a common measure applicable to both valued and devalued people.

Zola (1972, p 489) criticises the view that medicine's diagnostic expansionism into social and human problems is good since it de-stigmatises the deviant or aberrant. No longer are problems religious, legal or moral but "therapeutic and objective". Moral character is determined by conformity, or otherwise, to the prescribed medical solution to the problem (Zola, 1972). As a constant feature of the paradigm of care, compliance is a central prescription of the medical and medico-psychological models. The 'designation of deviance' in late modernity derives increasingly from the judgements of medicine (Conrad and Schneider, 1980). Because social control is now a fundamental role of medicine, a similar social control and 'designation of deviance' attends palliative care through its medicalised expression.

Role system and obligations

As Lofland (1978) illustrates, 'the happy death movement' prescribes a way of dying. Alternative roles, behaviours and understandings are devalued in the very act of valuing a certain way of dying. Seale (1998, pp 177-8) discusses alternative scripts to the 'aware dying role' (Seale, 1998, p 173) of the 'revivalist' discourses (Seale, 1998, p 63, citing Walter, 1994) that are dominant in palliative care (Seale, 1998, p 5). This 'revivalism' "proposes an elevation of the (supposedly) private experiences of dying and bereavement, so that these are brought into the field of public discussion" (Seale, 1998, p 4). The 'aware dying role', in which the dying "hero" is engaged in "emotional labour" (Seale, 1998, p 92), is important for understanding the prescriptions imposed and valued by palliative care culture. Both Lofland (1978) and Seale (1998) acknowledge that the socialisation of individuals limits their power to resist cultural scripts.

Saunders (1977, 1996) stresses that the hospice must provide the freedom for each individual "to have his/her own way of dying" (Saunders, 1977, p 164). Where she does acknowledge the possibility of converting individuals' ways of dying to the way of palliative care, for example by St Christopher's Hospice having a Christian basis, she implies that a proper openness in interpersonal interaction can circumvent these potential problems (Saunders, 1977). However, if unintentionally or intentionally prescription does take place, it is not simply the individuals in the organisation that are at fault, but also broader organisational forces that conform individuals to organisational culture. Saunders applies this very logic when using instances of residents following their own cultural scripts rather than those of St Christopher's Hospice to indicate that the hospice itself and its philosophy respect individual differences. Her examples of residents maintaining their non-Christian faith are used to confirm the hospice's acceptance of all faiths, not just by individual staff but also by organisational ideology or policy as a whole (Saunders, 1977). Interestingly, these examples are not seen as instances of residents' tenacious resistance to the dominant prescriptions of hospice culture.

Research, for example House (1993, cited in Franks, 1999, p 54), suggests problems in the uptake of palliative care services by various cultures and illness types may be due to services' failure to appreciate diversity with respect to culture and also non-cancer illness experiences (Franks, 1999, p 54). The distinction between failing to appreciate diversity and prescribing conformity is nominal. Seale (1998) also examines the relationship between the cultural scripts of palliative care and its exclusivity concerning disease groups, as well as examining cultural variations in dying scripts.

The expression of resistance or dissatisfaction by service users is problematic in palliative care because of the connection with gratitude and compliance and the social approval of palliative care as an institution. Wilkinson (1999a, p 100) notes that the "reluctance of the recipients of [all types of] care to express negative answers is well documented". Fear of punishment, for example by receiving less or no service, or being seen as ungrateful may be involved here. Small and Rhodes (2000) raise some issues around coercion and the difficulty of empowerment in the palliative care context, and also, citing Pearson (1995), state: "user involvement is only welcome when it conforms with what the professional wants to hear" (Small and Rhodes, 2000, p 215).

Although only relatively recently confirmed in palliative care by Cohen et al (1996, cited in Wilkinson, 1999a, p 98), respondents agreeing with positively framed statements and disagreeing with negatively framed statements has been more broadly studied as 'acquiescence' by Rouget and Harris (1994, pp 11-12), with respect to people with an intellectual disability. Rouget and Harris (1994) are interested in examining how staff ensure compliance by intentional and unintentional manipulation using various means, including questioning and other less overt cues. Cultural variations in questioning and non-verbal cues, not to mention in values, understandings and beliefs, raise significant challenges for palliative care to step beyond its Anglo-Saxon cultural expression, as Kanitsaki (1998) and Prior (1999a, 1999b) indicate. Wilkinson (1999a, p 98) verifies one element of the dynamics of acquiescence described by Rouget and Harris (1994) in noting that during face-to-face interactions the pressure to acquiesce may be increased. Citing Glickman (1997), Wilkinson (1999a, p 99) also notes the rarity of criticism of palliative care due to its high social approval.

These more subtle forms of obligatory responses required by palliative care as a specific cultural form have only begun to be explored. These critiques have arisen chiefly from investigations of the multicultural perspective, for example Gunaratnam (1997); Kanitsaki (1998); and Prior (1999a, 1999b). Gunaratnam (1997) stresses the need to reorient discussion away from culture and back to the exercise of power by the dominant culture. In commenting on cultural reductionism, she notes that "dehumanising themes are also interlaced with romanticised conceptualisations" (Gunaratnam, 1997, p 177). That romanticisation can be involved in the process of dehumanisation is critically important and new to palliative care.

Wolfensberger (1972, 1975) explains that romantic idealisation of devalued people is a major way to operationalise their social devaluation. To paraphrase Seale (1998), a central script of 'revivalist discourse' is the romantic, idealised role of the dying hero engaged in emotional labour and an intimate revival of the social bond. Wolfensberger (1972, 1975) specifies the historical role of the 'holy innocent' or 'eternal child' as the stereotypical idealised devalued role. A clear example of the imposition of this devalued role on a whole class occurs in the infantilisation of older people. Wolfensberger (1972, pp 22-5) gives numerous examples where 'holy innocents', by virtue of their condition, that is, their deviance alone, are perceived as very special to God and society. By association, so are those organisations and individuals who care for such people. That this kind of romantic idealisation has not been identified as a tool for devaluing people who are dying in palliative care is not surprising since its religious ethos implies that only goodness can be at work in such idealisation.

Saunders' assertion that hospice is not a building but a philosophy, able to be applied in any setting is a key belief that supports the idealisation of palliative care. This statement, reiterated by many, is now palliative care dogma. This dogma assumes that a programme or philosophy of care and the context in which it is delivered are separable. Conceiving of a programme of care in this decontextualised way assumes that a programme, philosophy or ethos can somehow transcend the context in which it is applied. The same error is involved when the religious ethos in palliative care is believed to be able to transmute palliative care's institutional, medicalised and professionalised organisation into a non-institutional, demedicalised and deprofessionalised organisation or type of care, while retaining all the core elements that enable institutional organisation, that is, primarily the religious and medical institution itself.

Saunders' dogma appears true because it is unarguable. It is unarguable because the proposition is tautologically constructed. A programme of care can never be a building, and vice versa. Or, since a philosophy or general programme of care contains, by definition, the specific case of that programme of care as it is applied in any particular setting or context, the dogma cannot be false. The tautology works or, that is, appears to hold some meaning by confounding the level of values or ideas with the practical level. While the hospice ethos or idea, being that which contains hospice values, can be applied anywhere, when it is applied it ceases being an ethos, set of values or idea and becomes a contextualised practice or a specific, context-bound instance of that idea. The irrefutability of Saunders' dogmatic assertion serves to confound criticism by virtue of an apparently indisputable, yet false, logical authority. The dogma elevates hospice to a rectitude beyond question.

Furthermore, the dogma constructs palliative care as a uniquely and qualitatively different way of caring to any other, when really any type of care, if it is genuine care, is "love in action" to use Bradshaw's (1996, p 412) term for the hospice ethos. Connor (1998, pp 111-14) discusses palliative care's belief in its uniqueness referring to this belief as the "arrogance of palliative care". The frequent identification of palliative care as a 'special' way of caring demonstrates the widespread belief in this construction. In any case, as Wolfensberger's (1998, pp 108-11) concept of model coherency explains, programmes of care and their contexts or applications should aim for a mutual coherence.

Street (1998, p 73) asserts that "many hospitals-in-the-home [programmes] ... create a clinic in the home rather than allowing the normal home routines to prevail". Medical care is not a hospital; institutional care is not an institution. These are philosophies or programmes of care that can be applied in any setting. Neither case denies or disproves that the hospital or the institution is the most extreme form and restrictive environment in which medical or institutional care is applied. The hospice dogma does not disprove or deny the fact that a hospice is an institution with all the devaluing negative effects of any institution of care. The institutional approach to palliative care is not confined to a building, the hospice, but rather resides within the palliative care philosophy or conceptualisation itself.

This widespread definitional obfuscation or unintelligibility in palliative care hides devaluing practices intrinsic to institutional programmes of care that are masked as good by the dogma's attribution of an extra-special uniqueness to palliative care. Although the unintelligibility involved in the concept of palliative care is unhelpful, there remains an inescapable problem concerning its religious ethos. This, or any other, ethos is no guarantee at all of protection against institutional abuses and devaluation, as the history of religious institutions demonstrates. As well as this fact being demonstrated in the history of medical hospitals and asylums, the almost daily reports of abuse and neglect in all sorts of institutions of care prove that the ethos of care itself is also no guarantee against devaluation. Wellard (1996, p 57, cited in Street, 1998, p 73), states that institutional care in the home is able to occur because nurses work within the "medical, physiological and technological discourses" that enable nurses to conform individuals to a way of caring that fosters compliance. And it could be added that nurses do so unconsciously generally and, therefore, independently of any religious ethos that they may consciously espouse or any programme of care, such as palliative care, that they may consciously apply based on such an ethos.

The hospitalisation of dying in the second half of the 20th century, which was part of the reason for the development of palliative care, remains significant (Backer et al, 1982). "Well into the 20th century the majority of deaths occurred in domestic homes ... [but] by the mid-1960s, two-thirds of all deaths in Britain occurred in hospitals or other places caring for the sick, and by 1989 this had risen to 71 per cent with only 23 per cent of 'home deaths'" (Field and James, 1993, p 8). Although 90% of time in the last year of the life of a person who is dying is spent at home (Franks, 1999, p 52, citing Neale and Clark, 1992), the proportion of home deaths has not increased (James and Field, 1992; Field and James, 1993; Field et al, 1997). A US report in 1988 stated that 80% of "the 2 million Americans who die each year do so in hospitals" (O'Connor, 1995, p 53). Since inpatient services represent authority, respectability and status, as well as ultimate expertise, they tend to exclude or marginalise alternative services, such as those centred on the home. Not surprisingly then, the existence of inpatient palliative care beds tends to decrease the numbers dying at home (Robbins, 1998, p 111; Mor and Hiris, 1983, cited in Bosanquet and Salisbury, 1999, p 38; Naysmith, 1999, p 172). And "it is increasingly difficult to prevent patients from being admitted to hospital or hospice for terminal care" (Naysmith, 1999, p 172).

The hospice or specialised inpatient palliative care unit needs to collect sufficient numbers of dying people together in order to allow research and teaching, just as the hospital collects people with the same conditions together. As McKnight (1977) indicates, institutional and professional agenda are not an apolitical, absolute good but an economic necessity for the service industry. In the paradigm of care, it was shown that the institutional agenda of medical care have not centred on the desire to advance medical science or provide care to those in need but around issues of economic reward, status and professionalisation, as well as those of intraprofessional rivalry. The poor and others with low social value have been institutionalised in the past in medical settings and suffered horrific abuse for the purposes of experimentation and teaching. Institutional care is the form of social organisation that is most useful for such agenda. A note of caution should be added, therefore, to the evidence of Komesaroff et al (1989, cited in Robbins 1998, p 119) who report that, in Australia, hospice inpatients were more likely to be non-professional, while home care patients were more likely to have had private insurance and be in professional or non-manual occupations. Citing Cartwright (1993) in addition to Komesaroff et al (1989), Franks (1999, p 52) indicates that "patients are more likely to die in hospital or hospice if elderly, single and poor". The serious risk to the welfare of people with an intellectual disability from hospice care in the US has been raised by Gibson (1984a, 1984b), Ellis and Luckasson (1984), Gordon (1984) and Wolfensberger (1984, 1992a).

From the paradigm of care it can be seen that a condition on continuing to receive care has been to comply, which in respect of medicalised care includes consenting to experimentation or to being used for teaching purposes. For people who are dying, the implicit pressure to consent in these areas is considerable. By contributing to the care of those that come after them, people who are dying can contribute to the heroic medical and medico-psychological conquest of the problems around dying. Especially, but not only, for people who may be seeking some kind of atonement prior to death, issues of consent regarding teaching and research, and compliance generally, in palliative care are shrouded in a coercive atmosphere.

Discussion of research in palliative care stresses the 'paramount importance' of ethical considerations, for example, Wilkinson (1999b, p 22). However, scant attention is given to ethical issues concerning freely given, informed consent, except where this relates to issues such as resuscitation or euthanasia. For example, in Wilkinson (1999b), ethical issues concerning consent seem to be not mentioned. Russon (1998) stresses that informed consent underpins palliative care and that some areas where this right can be infringed are: assessment of competence, respect for autonomy, coercion and manipulation, and inadequate information and time to deliberate. Randall and Downie (1999, p 242) question whether truly voluntary consent to research can ever be given by people who "may be in pain or discomfort, distressed or frightened". Bradshaw (1996, p 415) stresses the problem of the "real or imagined" obligation felt by patients to consent to research, since such obligation is part of the power inequality in the client–practitioner relationship. Randall and Downie (1999) define and stress 11 aspects to this power inequality. With such factors at work, all practitioners' suggestions, not just those regarding research, are open to influence by this obligation. While Gamlin (1998), for example, notes that choice, respect and control are important elements in dignity, these words have little meaning unless accompanied by an examination of how to enable the service user to resist the authority and prescriptions of palliative care culture and the professionals that embody it. Small and Rhodes (2000, pp 91–3) raise some of the difficult, related issues around choice, user involvement and empowerment in palliative care. After a considered and lengthy discussion, Randall and Downie (1999) conclude that it is unethical to define the user/family/carer as the unit of care because the benefit to the service user should take precedence over any benefit to the family/carer. When family/carer benefit conflicts with the user's benefit, especially in the vital cases of admission to and discharge from hospital/hospice, Randall and Downie (1999) conclude that the user's benefit should take precedence even if, in the case of discharge home, professionals judge the care at home would be inadequate.

Religious ethos

Gift of charity

The role of carer as one who can and should assist is defined in terms of religious duty and calling, especially in nursing. With respect to the development of the management of insanity, Porter (1992a, p 301), refers to this calling as the "sting in the tail that certain groups in society have a right and duty to improve others". This sting underlying care also presumes a reciprocal obligation on recipients of care to agree to accepting care. The ethical issues concerning consent in palliative care are deep and complex.

The correspondence between medicine and religion in modernity allows palliative care to marry its traditional religious ethos with the quasi-religious ethos of medical science. However, the attraction of the medical and medico-psychological discourses and their incorporation into palliative care has had serious negative repercussions according to the many authors who express concern over the erosion of the original palliative care ethos, for example, Bradshaw (1996) and Rumbold (1998, 1999). Bradshaw (1996) senses secularisation and a humanistic professionalism creeping in and specifies the return to the true religious ethos as the antidote. The solution to medicalising or bureaucratising or secularising palliative care appears to be to reassert hospice's true ethos. However, the true ethos of palliative care is variably defined, as the various emphases of Biswas (1993), Ahmedzai (1993) and Bradshaw (1996) show.

Saunders (1977) strips the true ethos to its bare bones. "We all ... must often say the wrong or hurtful thing, but as we keep coming for such simple errands we have the opportunity for a new beginning.... A true meeting between two people is a gift coming unbidden into the midst of such action" (Saunders, 1977, pp 164-5). Saunders (1977, p 175) recommends openness and complete simplicity as those things that allow the gift of meeting. It would seem, therefore, that no other quality or activity, such as espousing a religious ethos or even practice of a religious perspective, can cause a true meeting between people. This is consonant with the original conception of meeting, which derives from Buber (1961, 1970). The Christianised hospice ethos, "a genuine covenant meeting" in Bradshaw's (1996, p 413) words, appears some considerable way from Buber's meaning. Bradshaw (1996, p 418) also connects the hospice ethos to the concept of 'moral quality'. Her usage presumes that 'moral quality' exists in some more than others or in some but not in others, which implications distort Buber's understanding of the human being. Although Kaufmann (1976) acknowledges a 'love thy neighbour' resonance in Buber's thought, Kaufmann (1976) argues that Christian, chiefly Protestant, interpretations of Buber's notions are generally misleading, particularly the theological interpretations.

There is, therefore, some doubt about the authenticity or intelligibility of the hospice ethos especially in its Christianised formulations. Moreover, the Christian basis of hospice and the Christian missionary past of several prime movers in hospice care's development raise questions concerning the spread of this ethos internationally and the obligations prescribed by hospice as a movement. Evangelical fervour in some hospice rhetoric, for example Doyle (1995, p 387), illustrates hospice's missionary zeal. Questions concerning the missionary aspects of hospice assume greater significance when, for example, the 126-year history of Christian missionary activity in Japan has resulted in only a very low rate of conversion, about 1.5% of the population (Hinohara, 2000). However, with one exception all Japanese hospice units are Christian (Kellehear, 2005b, citing Ida et al, 2002).

In any case, the palliative care ethos conceived in Saunders' manner is interpersonal, or suprapersonal, and substantially ignores what occurs socially when an organisation avows a religious ethos. An organisation with a religious ethos brings with it a range of very significant effects and implications. Palliative care's true ethos, under Saunders' definition, involves an inscrutable meeting and a preparedness to continue to try to be simply open to this meeting, despite persistent error. The real problem, as has been said, is that an organisation's ethos cannot guarantee that the practices of the organisation are consonant with its ethos.

The original nursing ethos serves as an example with several parallels to palliative care. Godden (1997, p 185) refers to the "very uneasy compromise" at the heart of Nightingale's movement: "nursing was a paid occupation for women, but was constructed as a religiously inspired philanthropic vocation". In Australia, this tension enabled administrators and doctors to claim nursing an act of charity rather than an occupation (Godden, 1997). Nightingale increasingly espoused a Christian basis for nursing. Increasingly, the goodness of the religious ethos was used to mask the terrible state of nursing in her school (Godden, 1997). The problems, which for Nightingale lay in the individual faults of nurses, could be corrected by nurses being better Christians. Bradshaw (1996) suggests Nightingale fought against nursing registration, that is, against a professionalisation of nursing to ensure that the spiritual ethos of nursing rather than just its techniques would be preserved. For Saunders too, according to Bradshaw (1996, p 414), professionals' skills were only a means to an end, the establishment of the religious ethos of the hospice organisation.

The spiritual ethos of Nightingale nursing was individualistic, as in palliative care, thereby allowing the claim that it could be preserved through individual nurses putting the ethos into practice properly. The argument in both areas appears to be that since the ethos is the repository and source of an organisation's goodness, failure to live up to this ethos must be due to its erosion in the practice of individuals and in the philosophy of an organisation. Bradshaw (1996, p 418) has argued, with Nightingale it would seem, that the 'moral quality' of the staff determines how compassionate the organisation is. Even if moral quality could be discerned somehow, this approach, that the quality of staff determines the quality of the organisation, is as unrealistic as it is individualistic. Using staff of variable moral quality cannot be avoided, since Bradshaw's (1996) argument presumes different people have different degrees or types of moral quality. Despite the inappropriateness of judging the moral quality of any person, such determinations are impossibly biased, especially when every imperfect person making such judgements must themselves have some sort of deficiency in moral quality.

General organisational corruption cannot be avoided by seeking a high moral quality of staff or by any other individualistic means. All organisation simply decays. Entropy or chaos increases in all systems.

All organisations tend to converge toward an institutional mould or homogeneity, a process termed 'institutional isomorphism' (Di Maggio and Powell, 1983, cited in Paradis and Cummings, 1986, p 371). Following Di Maggio and Powell (1983), this conformity is not only an attempt to stabilise increasing disorganisation and uncertainty but also the result of pressure from existing institutions and from professionals to legitimise and standardise the organisation. Increasing decay, disorganisation and uncertainty, which are necessary concomitants to growth, cause organisational conformity given the underlying institutional and professional agenda. Admonishments to reassert a religious ethos in an organisation cannot ensure either that people will be moral or that organisational decay will be remedied, whether that decay is seen to come from medicalisation, secularisation, bureaucratisation or any other source. The religious ethos serves many purposes but none of these relate to ensuring that practice is consistent with organisational idealism. The history of the Nightingale experiment also illustrates these points.

Although specific matrons/nurses were a problem, which problem recurred necessarily, the corruption of the practice of the Nightingale ethos came about due to institutional pressure that sought to conform Nightingale nursing to the institutional, hospital system. "The defects in nurse training ... lie not in what was intended to be the 'Nightingale system' but in its abuse by the service needs of the hospital" (Baly, 1987, p 45). Palliative care nursing is another experiment that tries to rescue the idealism of nursing from its corruption by the institutional homogeneity demanded by the hospital system. Decay and institutional demands lead to homogeneity, which through repetition and lack of renewal leads to further decay, which leads to further organisational homogenisation. A prevailing conceptualisation of care becomes tightly constrained within a certain mould. Standards of care can then only be measured within the parameters defined by this institutional homogeneity, which further locks out critical renewal.

The development of Nightingale nursing also shows that the religious ethos cannot rectify decay and ensure that practice matches principle. Indeed Nightingale's case supports the opposite. A religious ethos appears to make it easier for decayed practice to continue because the goodness attaching to religion implies goodness rather than organisational decay, or evil, is at work. Bradshaw's (1996, p 418) statement that the heart of palliative care "depends on the moral quality of the people who work in it" implies that this is not the case for other 'less special' or 'less religiously inspired' vocations or human services. Such an implication invokes the very special goodness of the religious ethos. "The quintessential heart of palliative care is the kind of compassionate people involved in it" (Bradshaw, 1996, p 418). Mystification of palliative care, and death and dying, as something extra special is conveyed by such assertions and, by this means, the romantic idealisation of practitioners and recipients of care is affirmed.

Morality and meaning

Attempts by palliative care to re-emphasise the social, moral or religious dimensions of care are compromised by the de-emphasis of these same dimensions entailed in the medical and medico-psychological expression that dominates palliative care. For example, the more the suffering related to dying can be alleviated or managed, the more the religious and spiritual meaning of suffering becomes ambiguous, if only because Christ's tremendous physical suffering in dying ceases to resemble our own. This attendant de-emphasis of social, spiritual and religious meanings is another element in the dilemma facing reform that seeks to cause medicine to acknowledge moral issues, and to acknowledge its own role in defining a pseudo-morality that effectively sidelines moral issues. By incorporating modern medicine into palliative care's structure, the very elements that most challenge religious, social and moral explanations of the world are introduced into the core of palliative care. A self-contradiction becomes situated at the centre of palliative care because it seeks moral and religiously inspired reform of medical practice, which in turn sidelines moral and religious questions and perspectives. MacIntyre (1985, cited in Bradshaw, 1996, p 418) notes the compromised religious meaning of suffering in palliative care under the medical and medico-psychological models, whose values of "aesthetics, therapeutics and managerialism" rob people of the "confrontation with truth" that is death, according to Bradshaw (1996, p 418). Street and Kissane (1998) also note the compromised relevance and meaning of suffering as an attendant effect of modern palliative care.

With the place of suffering problematic in palliative care, its responses to the deep purpose and significance of suffering can reduce to a fatuous sentimentality or religiosity of the kind derided by Lofland (1978, p 101). Robbins (1998) unintentionally reveals this tendency towards a reduction to sentimentality, and also reveals the contradictions in palliative care that, in part, give rise to it.

> At the end of the day, dying is often a sad and distressing
> time for all concerned and palliative care does not change

that. Palliative care can help to anaesthetise the pain of biological death, facilitate acceptance of the void of social death, and offer company to the individual in his or her quest for the philosophical, existential or spiritual meaning of death (Robbins, 1998, p 146).

It seems difficult to maintain that palliative care can help so much in these many critical areas, and yet not radically change the sadness of dying and the distress dying can cause, not to mention, in the process, changing the spiritual meaning of suffering and death, especially with respect to Christianity.

Care of the body, care of the soul

The integrated age-old care of the body and soul becomes in modernity a compartmentalised collection of needs of the body and the rationality of the mind. Saunders' (Saunders and Baines, 1983, pp 14, 43-50) idea of 'total pain' attempts to draw together again the dimensions of a person that have been separated. The idea of the management of 'total pain' implies the idea of the management of the total need. The team approach to palliative care is a necessary outcome of this attitude, as Illich (1977, p 26) stresses in relation to healthcare generally. The rights and power of the citizen to choose what needs are managed are compromised under this approach (Illich, 1977; McKnight, 1977; Zola, 1977). Palliative care advocates client self-determination and client-directed care yet its structures, such as the interdisciplinary team, tend to compromise these goals.

The shift from patient-centred to object-centred medical cosmologies (Jewson, 1976), which includes the hospital becoming medical workshop, allowed the decision-making power in care to shift from the patient to the doctor and the hospital. Object-centred medical cosmologies emphasise the body as a visible conglomerate of parts as the central fact of the process of care. The medico-psychological cosmologies likewise somatise, individualise and objectify the soul or mind as being revealed by deviant behaviours, issues, problems, symptoms or biochemistry of the brain.

Palliative care imports much of the object-oriented cosmology of medicine not only via its medical and medico-psychological concepts but also via its importation of wide-ranging hospital/medical structures, processes and terms. Palliative care teams comprise the same personnel as the hospital, that is, doctors, nurses, social workers, pastoral care workers, allied health workers and volunteers. With the importation of key aspects of the hospital/medical model into palliative care comes the decision-making power of the hospital as institution and the whole symbolic meaning of the hospital, and an institution in general. Object-oriented principles oppose person-centred principles, as Boschma (1997) notes in discussing the attempts of holistic nursing to balance the object-oriented medical influence in US hospitals. The interrelationship between doctors' and nurses' roles and, more importantly, the symbolic implications of these roles are fundamental features of the medical model that, therefore, change only very slowly. Doctors and nurses mean medicine, illness, hospital, authority, care towards cure and a hierarchical, paternalistic role system. The ongoing struggle for nurses to act as autonomous professionals alongside doctors, discussed for example by Kuhse (1997), demonstrates that the symbolic and practical role definition and interrelationship between doctors and nurses is not easily shifted. In palliative care, an holistic person-centred approach to care attempts to moderate object-oriented medicine, yet imports extensive medical and medico-psychological influences into its organisation and practice.

Philanthropic connections

Self-interest

The state's formal role in care brings with it a displacement of the stigma of charity. Philanthropically funded care is charity. Recipients of care have been demonised in the past as burdens of charity. Any voluntary and philanthropic involvement in hospice and palliative care carries these implicit messages.

Clark and Seymour (1999, p 135) stress the role of philanthropy in the growth of hospices and point out that founding a hospice was "a visible sign of care within the community". Philanthropy has been a key aspect of hospice care's development, which Douglas (1992) regrets. Douglas (1992, p 579) is not just annoyed by the holier-than-thou image of hospice (in Britain), especially its "charity balls [and] committee loads of duchesses", he is perplexed that collective dying in "agreeable, secluded little places ... amid leafy glades" is thought to be a good thing, as Clark (1993, pp 173-4) notes. For the purposes of philanthropy, the validity or otherwise of this crucial charge is immaterial. The philanthropic model works to the advantage of philanthropists, via personal rewards, as well as to the advantage of the institutions founded by philanthropists, so that both can enjoy the social rewards attending institutional expression, such as authority, status, respectability and the maintenance of the 'gift relation'.

For Douglas (1992), palliative care, its staff, supporters and institutions, already enjoy too much status, authority and respectability, as implied by his article's sarcastic title, 'For all the saints'. Perhaps, as he claims, philanthropy has served its purpose as far as hospice care is concerned. Once the authority, charitableness and goodness of palliative care from its original religious and philanthropic connections has been subsumed under that of the medical context, philanthropy for hospice specifically can be of little service to palliative care's institutional needs. However, palliative care's saintly image can still very much serve the self-interest of philanthropists. The state, as modern philanthropist, and global corporations, from fast food chains to pharmaceutical companies, can imbue themselves with the goodness of the aura of palliative care by associating themselves with it. The goodness attending palliative care, where the social approval is almost total and an idealised heroism and intimacy go hand-in-hand, conveys an absolute commitment to people and to social responsibility. Such an image can be bought by few means other than philanthropic support for palliative care and related cancer services.

Privilege versus right

Philanthropic and voluntary involvement in palliative care confirms the archetypal notion of care as a privilege or gift. Equality is excluded by a philanthropic component in care and its 'gift relation' (Porter, 1989). For example, while a voluntary workforce may be interpreted as enhancing equality of status through deprofessionalisation, voluntary labour denies equality by providing services in a way that is only considered appropriate for devalued classes of people. Deprofessionalisation of medical or corporate services is not going to happen, but deprofessionalisation of care for people who are dying or older people or other devalued classes is a very real possibility, if not a current reality. Unionised labour understands well the devaluation of existing workers, and their product, that is involved in using a voluntary labour force. Doyle (1995) asserts that blurred team role boundaries are not appropriate, at least between professional and volunteer. "It is difficult, if not impossible, to employ many of them [volunteers] appropriately in direct patient care when at the heart of palliative care there has to be continuity, high-quality communication, and professional cohesion" (Doyle, 1995, p 382). Field and Johnson (1993, pp 206-13) examine some of the problems associated with a voluntary labour force. Especially since palliative care has significant philanthropic connections, voluntary labour magnifies the negative implications associated with philanthropy and care.

When the social context of the voluntary sector is considered, it seems difficult to argue that the effects of using volunteers are to equalise status, deprofessionalise and instil a sense of community. The central effect of using volunteers involves the perpetuation of negative social perceptions regarding the value of the people serviced by volunteers. In Britain, one quarter of all volunteers work in health and social welfare (Lynn and Smith, 1992, cited in Field and Johnson, 1993, p 204). The characteristics of the voluntary workforce combine several socially devalued attributes: predominantly female, non-working, middle-aged or older, unpaid, and working casual/few hours (Field and Johnson, 1993, pp 204, 207). The use of labour with significant devalued characteristics to help service a devalued group entrenches and intensifies social devaluation of that group, by juxtaposition and the transference effect of negative stereotypes (Wolfensberger, 1998). In Britain at least, volunteers are also predominantly white, more religious than the general population, and are more affluent, indeed from the two uppermost social groups (Field and Johnson, 1993, p 204). Although these characteristics are valued, voluntary palliative care labour, at least in Britain, has a definite religious flavour and overtones of the philanthropic gestures of the affluent classes towards the recipients of care.

Part Two
Palliative care and social devaluation

FOUR

Social Role Valorisation

Introduction

Originally religious approaches and the organisation of religious institutions dominate the landscape of care. When modern medicine and science supplant religion in political and social influence, the paradigm of care becomes dominated by medical approaches and the medical institution. In this way, the social devaluation of people who receive care is established and perpetuated by this paradigm, of which palliative care is a part. Palliative care, therefore, must express the social devaluation of people who are dying. An examination of the ways social devaluation operates in palliative care requires a theoretical tool that can analyse the process of social devaluation. The theory known as Social Role Valorisation (SRV) – "a high order concept for addressing the plight of societally devalued people and for structuring human services" (Wolfensberger, 1998, p i) – describes how social devaluation operates. This theory also identifies people who are dying or chronically ill as one of a number of classes at risk of social devaluation. SRV is, therefore, an appropriate theoretical framework to use to assess social devaluation in the palliative care system.

By eliminating the ways in which devaluation is perpetuated in palliative care, a new palliative care paradigm can be created where palliative care's organisation and practice more closely match its ideals. SRV theory can be used to guide this construction. This chapter introduces SRV and demonstrates its relevance to palliative care.

This chapter begins by examining, with respect to social devaluation, the key alternative frameworks to the conventional conceptualisation of palliative care. SRV is then defined, and the case is made for the suitability of SRV to analyse social devaluation in palliative care. The success of SRV and the key difference between the challenges in the disability sector and those in the palliative care sphere are examined. The chapter proceeds to address the existing criticism of SRV most relevant to palliative care and moves on to summarising the 10 core themes of SRV with some reference to the palliative care context.

Alternative frameworks

Besides the overarching tension concerning the compromised meaning of suffering and death, which is explored in Chapter Seven, there are three significant tensions in palliative care: first, the tension between some kind of primitive palliative care and Saunders' modern, professional religio-medical version; second, the tension between a perceived creeping medicalisation of palliative care and Saunders' original religio-medical ethos; and third, the tension between the nursing/medical and psychosocial/spiritual domains and their practitioners. Although not specifically discussed, various elements of these tensions are raised in later chapters. For example, Chapter Six discusses the vast scope of palliative care nursing practice, which reflects and intensifies the considerable tension between the nursing/medical and psychosocial/spiritual domains in palliative care. Chapter Five introduces the specialist-generalist dilemma, which reflects the tension between ideas about a primitive deprofessionalised palliative care and the utilisation of a specialised team of professionals. The two key alternative frameworks discussed shortly are also a reflection of these three fundamental tensions and the root contradiction in Saunders' conceptualisation from which they derive.

Defining palliative care within a medical context, as a health or aged care service, constructs dying as an abnormality or 'illness' with terminal care, at least, being managed in some sort of healthcare institution. Clark and Seymour (1999, pp 157-8) refer to several studies confirming that hospital admission in the last days of life is an increasing trend. SRV literature has long been critical of mechanistic approaches to community support that both establish institutional processes within community living arrangements and also work to deny social inclusion and participation, as Taylor (2005) indicates. Policy frameworks in community care in the health and social care sectors are shifting in a number of countries. For example, a focus on partnerships and new understandings of care coordination in the UK since 1990 has paralleled some shift in UK palliative care discourse. Sociological and social work critiques of mechanistic approaches to community care have arisen, with some reference to its interface with palliative care (for example, Clark, 1993; Neale, 1993; Clark and Seymour, 1999; Thompson, 2002; Thompson and Thompson, 2005). These critiques discuss various new approaches, for example, a shift toward primary healthcare teams (Clark and Seymour, 1999) or an emphasis on cultural assets and social resources such as bereavement self-help groups (Riches and Dawson, 2000, pp 16-24, 121). However, these critiques do not identify that the root of mechanistic approaches in palliative care lies in its conceptualisation, which is inherently biomedical. Furthermore, the devaluation of people who are dying is not understood to be the fundamental, intrinsic, negative effect of Saunders' conceptualisation. Race (2004) comments on 2001 UK policy directions in learning disability towards 'partnership boards' and 'person-centred approaches' and questions whether such processes will lead to outcomes sought by SRV. Without an SRV-based understanding, policies, services and approaches that use high-sounding terms, such as 'empowerment', 'person-centred', 'coordination', 'planning' and 'choice', are necessarily applied in devaluing ways because devaluation is not understood as deeply embedded into the human service system and its social control functions.

Two alternative frameworks have pointed to the serious negative impact of the current medicalised conception of palliative care. The primary alternative framework is 'health-promoting palliative care' pioneered by Kellehear (1999), which defines palliative care within the context of a public health service, outside the whole medicalised conceptualisation of palliative care. Kellehear's (1999) concern is not so much to provide a critique of the conventional model but to lay out a new ground plan from which novel and non-medicalised approaches to palliative care can evolve. Since Kellehear's (2005a) expansion of his public health approach to loss, death and end-of-life care contains a critique of normalisation theory, his later work is examined in the section 'Criticism of SRV' in this chapter. Although by no means as expansive as health-promoting palliative care, a second alternative framework is proposed by Corner and Dunlop (1997). While this framework is not an entirely new way to conceive of palliative care, and is not presented as such, scrutinising the whole social construction of palliative care, as Corner and Dunlop (1997) recommend, could lead to a new conceptualisation of palliative care. Corner and Dunlop's (1997) understanding that the essential nature of the current conceptualisation of palliative care is inherently biomedical is of crucial importance.

Being the first and, until the present book, the only social model of palliative care, health-promoting palliative care emphasises that the social aspects to dying and palliative care involve far more than clinical nursing/medical and clinical psychosocial/spiritual care. Health-promoting palliative care seeks to enable communities to engage with death and dying in novel ways and evolve their own responses to death and dying. Its ingenuity lies in it side-stepping clinical medical constructions altogether by adopting the new public health paradigm, which has already been accepted and instituted in the healthcare field to some degree. If health-promoting palliative care can have the same impact as health promotion generally has had on healthcare approaches at large, then it will have made a significant contribution toward reducing the dominance of the biomedical conception of the current palliative care model.

Kellehear (1998, pp 2–3) is clearly very much aware of the fundamental problems attending the clinical, medical conception of palliative care, including the fact of devaluation (Kellehear, 1984, p 717). Corner and Dunlop (1997) explicitly discuss some of these root problems and bring into question several of Saunders' fundamental ideas underpinning conventional palliative care. Kellehear (1998, p 3) notes that conventional palliative care is predominantly a nursing/medical endeavour. To facilitate the empowerment of the person who is dying and their support networks, health-promoting palliative care tries to reduce this nursing/medical dominance by advising, for example, that peer support groups and other education sessions be led by non-medical personnel. While nurse-led clinics are seen as a key means to shift the biomedical emphasis under Corner and Dunlop's (1997) proposal, health-promoting palliative care understands, therefore, that such a solution can be, at best, only partial because nurses are archetypal components of the biomedical approach. This kind of insight is important from an SRV-based point of view and illustrates the broader perspective of social models like health-promoting palliative care compared to clinical models like that of Corner and Dunlop (1997).

"The biomedical model of care ... represents the whole construction of care, and is adhered to by all participants in palliative care, consumers and professionals alike" (Corner and Dunlop, 1997, p 291). The diagnosis of the cause of a symptom, as deriving from bodily or mental operations in the individual, determines the kind of intervention pursued (Corner and Dunlop, 1997, p 295). Corner and Dunlop (1997) go on to describe the biomedical model's features as: the assumption that physical symptoms are the predominant cause of suffering in dying; best management is achieved by establishing the root cause of symptoms and relieving these by modern pharmacological and other biomedical means; psychological, social and spiritual aspects to symptoms are important but only secondarily; objectifying the problem risks "depersonalisation and decontextualisation of the problem" and a denial of "chronicity, suffering, distress and meaning as part of the illness experience" (Corner and Dunlop, 1997, p 291).

Corner and Dunlop (1997, pp 292–3) suggest a radical reframing of palliative care centring on a "scrutiny of [the] construction of care (political, social, cultural, physical and emotional)" and a deconstruction of power relationships and problems. However, since it remains a clinical model, Corner and Dunlop's (1997) approach seriously underestimates the problem of how to facilitate this deconstruction and how to achieve such a comprehensive scrutiny of all aspects of palliative care. Corner and Dunlop's (1997) analysis proposes no systematic way of undertaking the comprehensive review they recommend.

Corner and Dunlop (1997) and health-promoting palliative care (Kellehear, 1999) do not identify social devaluation as the primary negative effect of the current palliative care conceptualisation. They possess no evaluative tool to determine how the medical model and their own models perpetuate social devaluation. Because of its broad reach, health-promoting palliative care, in particular, has the potential to institute new ways or exacerbate existing ways of devaluing people who are dying, as a later section of this chapter demonstrates regarding Kellehear's (2005a) recent development of the 'compassionate cities' approach. Without an evaluative tool to analyse social devaluation as the most potent and all-embracing negative effect of the social construction of palliative care and human services in general, efforts to redefine palliative care within a social or less-medical model can only perpetuate the devaluation of people who are dying. On the other hand, SRV is theoretically and specifically designed to assess, analyse and address social devaluation in systems.

Definition of SRV

The term 'Social Role Valorisation' is first used by Wolfensberger (1983) as a new formulation of his variant of the principle of normalisation. Nirje (1969), the formal founder of normalisation, defined the original rights-based view of normalisation as the principle that people with an intellectual disability have the right to experience the normal rhythm of the day, week and year; to experience variety and choice; to participate in normal activities; and to experience the normal developmental events in the life cycle that most people experience.

Normalisation's origins stem from 1951-52 in care for people with an intellectual disability in Denmark, where legislation was enacted in 1959 (Bank-Mikkelson, 1980; Wolfensberger, 1980). In 1967, legislation involving some normalisation principles also was enacted in Sweden. The (US) President's Committee on Mental Retardation commissioned the monograph by Kugel and Wolfensberger (1969), cited in Wolfensberger (1980, p 75). With chapters by Bank-Mikkelson

(Denmark), Nirje (Sweden) and Wolfensberger (US), this monograph forms the basis of all future developments in normalisation.

Although originally sharing with Nirje (1969) a focus on rights (Wolfensberger, 2002, p 253), and the conditions reflecting these rights, Wolfensberger progressively saw that focusing on outcomes was inadequate because process, at all levels, needed to be addressed (Wolfensberger, 1980, p 79). Brief and informal definitions among SRV proponents amounted to saying that SRV involved 'using culturally valued means to achieve culturally valued ends'. The idea of the sheltered workshop serves to explain this critical insight concerning the coherence between means and ends. While the culturally valued outcome of the right to employment can be achieved by providing employment in sheltered workshops, since this is not the culturally valued means of employing (valued) people, the overall effect of such an approach is to increase social devaluation. The incoherence between means and ends corrupts both, serving to increase the overall devaluation effect.

In the same way, day care centres in palliative care increase devaluation because they do not use culturally valued means to achieve the culturally valued ends they seek, such as recreational, educational or social goals. Day care centres replace the ways that valued people engage in these activities with substitutes for devalued people, that is, 'dying people' only. The incoherence between means and ends creates a strange juxtaposition that makes the activity, setting and goal more peculiar. It is not surprising that, in response, this strangeness or abnormality tends to be cloaked in romantic idealisations about the 'very special and caring' nature of the activity, setting, goal and people involved.

Danish and Swedish models could retain the idea of a benevolent institution since the generalised processes of devaluation that drive social responses, including service system processes, were not central to Scandinavian approaches. However, Wolfensberger sees an inherent dependency and deindividualisation in institutional models of care that denies the real value of living. McKnight (1977, 1995) sees a similar dependency as the critical feature of modern human service systems. For Wolfensberger, the service system process known as institutional care fundamentally contradicts the principle of normalisation. Since no valued person would choose to live in institutional care, unless society restricts the availability of other support options, and since certainly the most valued in society would never subject themselves to institutional care, it is a devalued means, for devalued people only. Institutional care, no matter how benevolent or caring, can never be valued living with the rights, responsibilities, risks and opportunities enjoyed by many.

Sociological use of the term 'normalisation' refers to making social characteristics, such as ageing, death and dying, socially normative. Normalising death and dying refers to a social inclusion or integration of death and dying as culturally normative experiences, as experiences that are included and integrated within social norms rather than excluded by them. Psychological usage, for example in 'normalising grief reactions', reduces normalisation's meaning to apply to clinical circumstances.

Wolfensberger (1980) understands that people are denied culturally normative experiences because their behaviours, attitudes and roles are not culturally normative. The processes of both social devaluation and social valuation revolve around the same "feedback loop" (Wolfensberger, 1998, p 75) between roles, expectancies and perceptions. This feedback loop is inescapable and used by all of us all the time in social interaction. All of us are socialised into ways of behaving according to cultural norms and use this knowledge in every social interaction in order to present ourselves to the world and engage it. SRV theory explains how to use the knowledge of the feedback processes known as "role expectancy" and "role circularity" (Wolfensberger, 1998, p 106) to advantage people at risk of being excluded because their behaviours, attitudes or roles are culturally devalued by the norms of the dominant culture.

The most recent definition of SRV is "the application of what science can tell us about the enablement, establishment, enhancement, maintenance and/or defense of valued social roles for people" (Wolfensberger, 1995, cited in Osburn, 1998, p 7). "It is very important that they [people] be seen as occupying valued roles, because otherwise, things are apt to go ill with them." And others are more likely to grant the "good things of life" to people who occupy valued roles (Wolfensberger, 1998, p 58).

Williams offers the following brief summary of SRV theory:

> The process of devaluation consists of perceptions of people as being in negative social roles – eg as nuisance, sick person, object of pity, eternal child, danger to society – with negative consequences for the person – eg loss of opportunity, rejection, segregation, lack of choice, poverty, risk of abuse. The consequences are mediated through social processes of restriction, control, scapegoating, de-skilling and negative imaging. The response of an individual or group to this

> devaluation may reinforce the negative social perception
> of them in a highly negative and damaging feedback loop.
> SRV seeks to break into this process ... so that the process
> is reversed into one of social valuation rather than
> devaluation. The achievement and maintenance of valued
> social roles for people is sought. (Williams, 2004,
> Introduction)

According to SRV theory, the processes of social devaluation and its
remediation are universal, as are the processes of social valuation. SRV
principles, therefore, apply to any group at risk of devaluation, or to
any valued people. In asserting that (his version of) normalisation is
almost unique in its "universal applicability to human services",
Wolfensberger (1980, p 88) states: "all the bad things that happen to
devalued people are derived from a relatively small number of
universally recurring dynamics; and all the constructive things that
should be done can similarly be based on a relatively small number of
principles". When a person, group or class is cast into one or more of
10 devalued roles or stereotypes, social devaluation has begun. These
10 devalued roles, described by Wolfensberger (1972, 1975, 1998),
portray the devalued person as:

- other, alien
- sick, diseased organism, contagion
- the object of dread/menace, sinner
- the object of pity
- the burden of charity
- the object of ridicule
- the holy innocent
- child (eternal child, once again a child)
- sub-human or non-human organism, insensate object
- dying, already dead, as good as dead, useless.

Our colloquial vocabulary concerning devalued people is full of
derogatory words, expressions and images that encapsulate these
devalued roles. The dynamics of social valuation/devaluation operate
across all levels of the social system (Wolfensberger, 1972, 1998).

All societies distinguish between valued groups and devalued or
deviant groups (Wolfensberger, 1992a, pp 4, 8; 1998, p 5). "In every
society certain persons are unwanted. Their identity varies from time
to time, from place to place" (Szasz, 1994, p 7). In commenting on the
universality of social stratification according to power, privilege and

status, Wolfensberger (1992a, p 4) states "oppression almost inevitably goes with stratification, and since stratification goes with human societies, all human societies contain at least some elements of oppression, and usually a great deal". As a key institution within modern society, the human service system must both reflect and propagate dominant social values and social stratification. The necessary corollary, which is not acknowledged by and large, is that human services must reflect and propagate the dominant culture's judgements about what is deviant and what therefore should be devalued. This latter function of human services must be seen as intrinsic to their nature rather than assuming that, because human services aim to care, they are different or less flawed than other social systems.

Since positive expectations surround valued social roles, by manipulating the contexts of people at risk of devaluation these positive expectations can be made to increase. By this method, the kinds of roles available to and imaginable by devalued groups can be expanded. The mere presence of previously devalued classes in valued roles shifts these expectations markedly and, thereby, shifts the definition of what is socially valued. Today, since, for example, some African Americans assume valued social roles in the US government, an African American US president becomes a possibility, albeit a remote one due to the depth of the social devaluation of African Americans, as Elliot (1996) laments. The mere existence of African Americans in highly valued roles promotes and reflects a shift in what is socially valued, and also a positive shift in what is expected of and imaginable for *every* African American.

Success of SRV

The international penetration of normalisation and SRV illustrate their credibility. SRV principles have spread internationally and underpin legislation in many countries in the field of disability services and to a much lesser extent in the mental health and aged care sectors. Since social integration into normal communities is a major aim of SRV, its principles are able to be extended readily to fields with a community living emphasis. Deinstitutionalisation, without being underpinned by SRV theory and the further community support and development it advises, is being abused as a way to reduce government expenditure and, in effect, dump people into communities. Flynn and Nitsch (1980), Flynn and Lemay (1999) and Johnson and Traustadóttir (2005) provide assessments by various authors about the success of SRV and some of the key problems that remain.

One of SRV's basic principles, that devalued people should be physically integrated into society, has become widely accepted within the field of disability. The deinstitutionalisation of people with an intellectual disability has created in several countries the expectation that normal housing should be available for all people with an intellectual disability. For example, residential services using ordinary housing are the preferred model now in Britain for people with a disability (Alaszewski and Wun, 1994, p 171). The problems of the staged supported living systems like the community residential unit/ group home model, mentioned, for example, by Taylor (2005) regarding the US, and Gardner and Glanville (2005) regarding Australia, have for some time been identified by a number of services and remedied, particularly in the US. Jay Nolan Community Services (JNCS) is one such service (JNCS, 2006). "In 1992, JNCS began changing the way it provided services. The organisation closed its group homes and began providing supports to people to enable them to live in their own homes, have jobs, and participate in other valued activities" (JNCS, 2006).

As already mentioned, SRV's measure of success is the "enablement, establishment, maintenance and/or defense of valued social roles" (Wolfensberger, 1995, cited in Osburn, 1998, p 7), and, as a corollary, this success also entails eliminating or avoiding entry into devalued roles. The intellectual disability services sector has proven that:

- closing all institutions throughout a (chronic care) service sector is feasible and sustainable; and that
- physical integration of people into the community does not lead to their social integration without further eliminating quasi-institutional settings and approaches, such as group homes, and without further individualising supports.

The second point indicates that valued social roles are not enabled or established simply by people living in ordinary housing in the community. Devalued people do not automatically become valued members of the community solely through living in the community. On deinstitutionalisation, people with an intellectual disability, for the most part, had never experienced physically living in the community, much less experienced a valued social role. Instead people had been subjected to a lifetime of constant deprivation, humiliation and abuse. The challenges to enabling inclusive lives through valued social roles were, therefore, considerable, and remain so, although great successes have been achieved (for example, various authors in Johnson and

Traustadóttir, 2005; JCNS, 2006; Macomb-Oakland Regional Center, 2006).

The challenges for a deinstitutionalised palliative care system would be different and much less complex than in the disability sector. The central difference is that the vast majority of people who are dying will have led valued and socially integrated lives. As the critical example, the need to achieve non-institutional, socially integrated accommodation (that is, a home of one's own) will not be relevant since people who are dying will, for the most part, be already established in their own home. They will also already be established, or have been established, in non-institutional, socially integrated employment, relationships, education, recreation, community networks and so on. People who are dying, for the most part, will have valued histories.

Currently therefore, from an SRV-based perspective, success for palliative care means eliminating the devalued roles imposed by institutionalisation and maintaining the valued roles that already exist. The measures required to address social devaluation within the palliative care system are much more straightforward and readily achievable than the measures required within the intellectual disability sector. In palliative care, there will be little need to enable or create valued roles. The whole focus will be on maintaining existing valued roles, primarily that of home owner/occupier, and avoiding people entering devalued roles, via institutionalisation, institutional approaches to care and negative social imagery. Palliative care also has the advantage of knowing deinstitutionalisation is achievable and sustainable, and the advantage of having a model on which to base the deinstitutionalisation of palliative care and its future development. The question for palliative care is the same one that confronted the intellectual disability service system 30-40 years ago: to close all institutions of care and address the social devaluation they cause, or not?

Social devaluation of dying

The idea that death and dying, and so people who are dying as a class, are socially devalued has only been considered relatively indirectly in the palliative care literature. For example Kellehear (1990, p 12) asserts that "the growth of the view that death is a form of stigma" is one factor that has contributed to the 20th-century institutionalisation of dying in hospitals and nursing homes, and his study discusses some observations concerning the manifestation of the stigma experienced by people who are dying. Kellehear (1990, p 17, citing Baider, 1972, p 209) comments that "caught within medical definitions, hospital environments and the ideology of the sick role the dying are stigmatised as helpless and hopeless. They have no social identity and recognition other than those connected with their transitional status". Furthermore, Kellehear (1984, p 717) maintains that "the major sociological shift of the dying role, this century in contrast to all others, is this. Today the dying are second class citizens alongside drug addicts, convicts, alcoholics and disliked ethnic groups".

In contrast to the palliative care literature, Wolfensberger's (1998) work centres on the idea of devaluation and has specifically identified people who are dying to be a class at risk of social devaluation. He broadens the ideas of stigma and deviance and related sociological constructs by using the concept of devaluation. Devaluation can operate in any setting, not just within institutions, and operates via universal processes across all devalued classes. Although the ideas concerning the stigma around death and dying and the related idea of death as a modern taboo have become widespread, these ideas have been muddied by connecting them with the death–denying society hypothesis. This hypothesis distorts the meaning of these ideas by implying modern society chooses to ignore or cannot face death when the reality is very different, as Kellehear (1984), Walter (1991) and Seale (1998) show. Death as a commodity is enthusiastically embraced by the funeral industry (Kellehear, 1984, p 719). The pharmaceutical, medical and human service industries do likewise by their involvement in palliative care.

Rather than devaluation necessarily involving some kind of evil intent by society, although certainly devaluation can be motivated by evil, devaluation in its various forms is a functional device to express the worth of membership in society. Wolfensberger (1992a, pp 7-8) describes the usefulness of devalued classes to society and to individuals in society. The identity of group members and the security offered by the group is defined by who is 'in' and who is 'out'. The 'in' group asserts its status by giving privileges to its members and not to others. Status is bestowed on 'deviancy managers', that is, on people and organisations who deal with deviant people in a formal sense. And finally, deviancy allows 'scapegoating' or victimisation. Social tensions or problems are believed to be caused by the devalued class and so resolved by modifying or managing that class.

For example, Scitovsky (1984, p 606) warns of the "new ethical problems of major proportions" that medical care cost containment might involve unless the overall cost of medical care is examined rather than the costs of medical care for particular populations. There is "the very real danger of policies being formulated which would relegate very sick patients, and especially very sick elderly patients, to a 'terminal' group before their time to die has come" (Scitovsky, 1984, p 604). Containing the cost of care is likely to be targeted at devalued groups rather than rationalising costs across all sectors. Far from social devaluation assuming a denial of one class's existence, as in the death-denying society hypothesis, social devaluation assumes an aggressive acknowledgement of that existence by, for example, actively marginalising the social participation of that class via segregated environments, such as nursing homes, hospices or inpatient palliative care units.

The explosion of literature about death in the second half of the 20th century, noted by several authors as disproving the death–denying society hypothesis (for example Kellehear, 1984, p 715), as well as the explosion of hospice care in this period attest to an intensification of formal concern with and management of death and dying. If death and dying represent deviance to modern society, then such intensification is likely to represent a quickening in the dynamics of social devaluation. The hospitalisation of death hid death, part of the 'sequestration of mortality' to use Seale's (1998, p 3) term, and constructed dying as a phenomenon requiring a total institutional response. The increased profile of death in the latter half of the 20th century signified a shift that made death and dying more visible as social phenomena, and more rational and manageable as ideas and, later, as objects of palliative care management.

This book's perspective questions the suggestion that these kinds of changes represent an increasing acceptance or relevance of death and dying to modern society. It is far more likely that these changes merely signify a shift in social management response without affecting the underlying fact of social devaluation. Especially since hospice care itself centres on an institutional model of management, there seems little reason to suspect any radical shift in social attitudes or in the social organisation of care for people who are dying is taking place. Social devaluation is inherent in models of care with significant institutional expression. Although the deviance of death and dying may be relabelled by its 'hospicisation', just as previously it was relabelled as 'acute' illness by its hospitalisation, the underlying deviance designation remains, a point made by Conrad and Schneider (1980) in relation to deviance designation in general under modern medicalisation.

Wolfensberger (1992a, 1998) acknowledges people who are dying as one of the classes at risk of social devaluation. Just as ageing, which occurs to the vast majority, has become socially devalued in late modernity, the idea that dying has also become socially devalued or deviant is not unreasonable, if only because an increasing majority of people die in old age. Today, "ageing is also seen as a form of dying", as Kellehear (1990, p 55) asserts. Williams (2004) uses the term "dyingism" to name specifically the devaluation of the class of people who are dying.

Of the classes in western society that Wolfensberger (1992a, pp 33-4) states are apt to be or become socially devalued, those with particular relevance to palliative care are: "people who are terminally ill", "people who are severely and chronically ill", and "infirm elderly persons especially if they are poor". In his later work (Wolfensberger, 1998, pp 9-10) he reorganises the classification in this way:

- "those who are impaired in some way ..." (in this group are placed the chronically, severely and terminally ill classes);
- "those who are seriously disordered or unorthodox in their conduct or behaviour ...";
- "those who rebel against the social order ...";
- "the poor ...";
- "those who have very few skills or whose skills are not wanted or useful to society ...";
- "those who are unassimilated into the culture ..." (in this group are placed older people and the unborn/newborn classes).

SRV theory concerns all and any of these classes. Wolfensberger (1992a, pp 33-4) remarks that any combination of these groupings in one person multiplies the risk and degree of social devaluation. Since older people and chronically ill people are an increasing majority of those who die, death and dying in old age is an important example of this idea of 'double devaluation' and its compounding negative effects. Wolfensberger (1992a, 1998) comments that he has derived his classification of groups at risk of social devaluation by determining which groups' behaviours, images, values or attitudes conflict with those of the dominant culture in the West. Growing old has become devalued because the facts and symbols of ageing conflict with dominant social norms such as independence, youth, health and beauty. Following the pattern observed by Conrad and Schneider (1980), since growing old is a modern deviance the 'medicalisation of oldness' (McKnight, 1995, p 64) is a logical development. Palliative care can be considered part of this 'medicalisation of oldness'. Death and dying also conflict with modern social norms and embody symbolic challenges to modern values. Some of these values challenged by devalued groups are: the myth of materialistic individualism; the myth of "entitlement to whatever one wants"; and the "belief of quasi-religious proportions that affliction, suffering and hardship are evil, and that they can, must and will be eliminated, and by human efforts" (Wolfensberger, 1992a, pp 25-6).

Wolfensberger's (1992a, p 73) priority listing of the 10 human service settings where the lives of devalued people are most at risk, ranks "residential hospices for the dying" second only to abortion clinics/services (the unborn child is the class at risk). His ranking applies only to those US hospices that are a "branch of the nursing home business" (Wolfensberger, 1992a, p 74), which hospices he considers are "rarely anything like" St Christopher's Hospice (Wolfensberger, 1992a, p 74). He also specifies that the best thing about US hospice is that it extends care into people's homes (Wolfensberger, 1984, p 168). Wolfensberger (1992a) sees a "new genocide of handicapped and afflicted people" occurring in modern society. Gibson (1984a) expresses fears that hospice care might be used to institute a socially sanctioned eradication of devalued classes via euthanasia, for example. Concerning the care of older people, Doyle (1990, p 8) warns "we [the palliative care profession] may find ourselves looking after those of its [society's] members society does not find attractive" and must "ensure our work is not hijacked by those who would promote active euthanasia". These kinds of risks imply an ethical imperative for palliative care to become conscious of its devaluation of people who are dying.

Criticism of SRV

The major criticisms of normalisation and SRV can be found in Perrin and Nirje (1985), Baldwin and Hattersley (1991), Brown and Smith (1992) and Flynn and Lemay (1999). Flynn and Nitsch (1980) contain responses to the criticisms more specific to normalisation than SRV, for example, Wolfensberger (1980). In Flynn and Lemay (1999), some recent criticisms are addressed by Wolfensberger, such as that of the so-called 'social model of disability', a Marxist/materialist approach based on disability rights and ideas of oppression by dominant groups (Wolfensberger, 1999, 2002). Race (1999) offers an extensive survey and response to major criticisms of SRV. Race (2003) includes articles from Wolfensberger, which also clarify issues relevant to various criticisms. Shortly, Kellehear's (2005a) brief critique of normalisation with respect to end-of-life care is specifically considered in some detail, because it criticises various approaches adopted by the present book.

One of the key criticisms in the literature mentioned has particular relevance to the palliative care context because the criticism arises from the religious or moral stance that people should be valued in themselves. This criticism involves some sense that people should be valued not for their roles, but as they are, for their intrinsic worth.

Value people as they are

Palliative care seeks to value people as they are, in themselves, since this is a prescription of the religious ethos (for example, Saunders, 1977). Bayley (1991, p 89) quotes Wolfensberger's (1983, p 238) attitude that asserts that valuing people in themselves has "merit and validity" but is "almost totally ineffective in bringing about the desired goal" (that is, increased social valuation of the person). Race (1999, pp 148-9) teases out what Wolfensberger (1983) means. Race explains that the proposition to value people in themselves, as they are, is true and meritorious at the level of values. However, at the pragmatic level of social interaction, since no person can avoid making a whole host of conscious and unconscious judgements both positive and negative about others' behaviours, characteristics, attitudes and so on, the exhortation to 'value people as they are' has no practical meaning. In social reality, self-evidently people cannot be viewed as they are, since it is impossible to view people as if no social context surrounded them. We learn how to function as people in society by making countless judgements about our impressions of ourselves and others. At the practical level, a person is not separable from his/her roles. Only at the moral and abstract level is a person separable from his/her roles. Wolfensberger means that if a person values another, the *only* way the former can show it is through enhancing the latter's valued roles and/or reducing the latter's devalued roles.

Palliative care, because of its religious ethos, is quite properly bound to assert the 'value-people-as-they-are' proposition at the moral level. However, this position allows devaluation to be masked in practice, and implies that people and organisations espousing this value stance cannot, would not or do not devalue others. Thinking that we already do or can value devalued people, as they are, allows a whole host of devaluing acts to be mistakenly believed to be good and caring acts, as the tragic history of institutional care shows. Bayley (1991, p 89) comments that the class of people with an intellectual disability represent a "challenge to see what mentally handicapped people can reveal about ourselves and the society we live in". In the same way, the class of people who are dying can also be considered to be serving a similar social function as some sort of unwitting 'social conscience' or 'wise counsel'. The peculiar assumption is that society can somehow learn to value the function of the devalued class to reveal society's own prejudices, to challenge its materialism, intolerance, lack of compassion, or obsession with youth and beauty for example, when society itself has designated devalued status according to these very valuations. Society cannot contradict its own valuations, and will aggressively react to reinforce these existing values by further marginalising the devalued class and its challenge, whether actual or symbolic. That devalued people serve this function is self-evidently true, at the level of values, since devalued classes, by definition, challenge dominant social values. To suggest, however, that at the practical level devalued people serve this function, which occurs by virtue of their devalued characteristic alone, denies their conscious agency, or subordinates it to an imposed or overlaid greater purpose. A range of other devaluing implications is involved in ascribing this function to devalued people.

The following discussion uses Kellehear's (2005a) public health approach to explore common misunderstandings about devaluation in the 'value-people-as-they-are' argument that pervades palliative care. Kellehear (2005a) invokes a quasi-religious ethos of compassion and its absolute good. "[W]e must restore the idea and practice of compassion to its rightful place – at the very top of our public health priorities" (Kellehear, 2005a, p 163). This is indisputable, at the level of values. However, at the practical level, when trying to ensure such practice matches compassionate ideals, the difficulties from various sorts of devaluation are formidable, as Kellehear's (2005a) list of threats to developing 'compassionate cities' shows. Unless SRV theory informs approaches that do not exclusively and explicitly focus on devaluation issues, these approaches can only succeed in reproducing, in both standard and novel forms, the devaluation that denies the development of compassionate communities.

Kellehear (2005a) sees loss and death as "universal and normative experiences". He argues that loss and its suffering can serve to evoke empathy or compassion, since we all share loss in some form or other. Loss is a prefiguration, foretaste or symbol of death. People who are dying are at serious risk of devaluation (Wolfensberger, 1992a, 1998) because "[t]he violence and finality of death is an affront to everything we value ..." (Kellehear, 2005a, p 162). However, Kellehear (2005a) also implies that inequalities can be addressed by this same means of developing empathic identification among 'all people' based on the shared experience of loss. This is a variant of the value-people-as-they-are argument, as will be shown shortly. His argument tends to imply that 'all people' can be valued, including devalued people even though they occupy devalued roles, because we all share a sense of loss. Kellehear (2005a) does say devalued roles should be addressed, but his focus is intentionally skewed toward an abstract and amorphous 'all people' in order to try to awaken a sort of generalised appreciation of loss and compassion in communities.

The key problem with this argument is that it involves an effective imposition like the one mentioned previously. People who are experiencing, or have experienced, the most or deepest losses also happen to be the members of the most vulnerable and devalued groups. Devalued people have the role of unwitting 'social conscience' or 'wise counsel' effectively imposed on them for the benefit of others. Ironically, the loss of social status is imposed on devalued people and then the role of teaching society about the nature of devaluation and its multiple losses is further imposed on them in order to reform society's materialism, individualism, lack of compassion and so on. There seems little in this for devalued people especially since, in order to learn about loss for example, there is an added incentive to ensure that devalued people continue to embody the deepest losses. Devalued people have imposed on them yet another devalued, romantically idealised role as heroic battler against loss or as unwitting wise counsel for the benefit of us 'all', which means, in effect, all valued people.

Kellehear (2005a, p 162) explains that "the compassion we offer one another can only be equitable and unwavering if this arises from a genuine empathy". And he further states that "only by seeing ourselves in the other do we seriously take up the challenge of emerging from a narcissistic and inward-looking individualism" (Kellehear, 2005a, p 161). This heroic ideal involving an emotionally intimate empathy resembles the religious ethos of hospice, which is not surprising since "love in action" (Bradshaw, 1996, p 412) is just another way of saying compassion in action.

Although unarguable at the level of values, this ethos effectively imposes a romantically idealised role on people at risk of devaluation and devalues them as a result. Under this perspective, of necessity we unintentionally see the devalued characteristic first, whether it be dying, loss or disability, and see it always superimposed on the person, which is the exact opposite of what we intentionally try or hope to see. To value devalued people as they are, that is, as socially devalued, involves a contradiction that pretends it can deny or transcend the social reality of the devalued difference. The 'value-people-as-they-are' argument evokes the holy innocent devalued role in which the disability, dying, loss or other devalued characteristic is seen as special or holy, in and of itself – actually or virtually – because it teaches us to develop empathy, to confront our individualism, narcissism or materialism, or challenge some other dominant social value.

Additionally, trying to address devaluation by emphasising commonalities shared by 'all people' has no meaning at the practical level because devaluation consists, precisely, in a mindset that *must* see no relevant commonalities between the valued and devalued person. In fact, were a commonality to threaten to appear in a devalued person, the devaluing mindset has to see this appearance of commonality as the worst kind of difference. To the devaluing mindset, devalued people threatening to embody a commonality represents an arrogation by devalued people of a commonality that rightfully can only belong to the people doing the devaluing. For example, sadness in a devalued person *must* be seen by a devaluing mindset as weakness, incompetence, stupidity, sickness, selfishness, childishness, ingratitude and so on. The devaluing mindset *must* work tirelessly to distort every possible commonality into a difference, in almost deliberate disregard for glaring commonalities, chiefly human embodiment itself. Since the devaluing mindset cannot sufficiently appreciate the commonality of human embodiment itself, then the likelihood of the commonality of loss or suffering striking an empathic chord seem distant.

Kellehear (2005a) also offers a brief critique of normalisation theory. This critique is discussed in some detail at this point because it is the only critique of normalisation from within palliative or end-of-life care and because this critique raises questions about the approach of the present book, particularly concerning its effectiveness and reach. Kellehear's (2005a) own recommended strategies are used in the following discussion to illustrate the general problems with his critique and his 'value-loss-as-it-is' approach in relation to devaluation issues. Raising these problems is not meant to minimise the importance of his approach in broadening the restrictive clinical and medical idea of modern palliative care, but rather to seek to demonstrate the overarching importance and power of SRV as an analytical tool to disclose how social devaluation is embedded and hidden in social processes.

While Kellehear's (2005a) discussion of normalisation and SRV is broadly supportive of the approaches and objectives recommended by the present book, he sees some theoretical problems and, more importantly, significant limitations of these approaches in addressing the entire spectrum of end-of-life care. In specifying some of the common criticisms of normalisation, Kellehear (2005a, p 33), with virtually no discussion, assesses much of this criticism to be "valid", although these criticisms have been comprehensively addressed by SRV proponents over the past 35 years. These proponents, such as

Race (1999), would disagree with Kellehear's (2005a) assessment. Kellehear's (2005a) understanding of SRV concepts and their meaning appears confused in light of several of his explanations. As one example, Kellehear (2005a, p 32) seems to use the word 'passing' in reference to devalued people achieving an understanding of themselves, when 'PASSING' (Wolfensberger and Thomas, 1983) refers to a technical term for a detailed 42-criteria assessment tool of *services'* achievement of normalisation goals. The idea of devalued people passing or failing in their understanding "about which unnecessary features in their behaviour or attitudes are creating barriers from others" (Kellehear, 2005a, p 32) entails a set of convoluted misunderstandings about SRV theory.

However, Kellehear (2005a) correctly points to a community development emphasis as the key common ground between SRV-based approaches and public health approaches. Kellehear (2005a, pp 86-7), referring to Giddens, partly bases his approach on "Third-Way politics" and political and social understandings around participation, partnership and a revision of "our ideas about inequality and community as problems of social inclusion". Race (2004) examines some of these innovations in the UK, such as partnership boards, with respect to SRV and shows that, while these concepts and their principles appear to involve "SRV thinking", they prove, through the approaches corresponding to these principles, to misconstrue SRV goals and understandings particularly concerning the operative power of "the entrenched services system". Wolfensberger (2002) explains how high-sounding principles tend to embed devaluation more deeply and hide it in fashionable terms such as 'empowerment', 'autonomy' and 'choice', whose SRV-based understandings are notoriously abused especially by policy makers and the service system.

For example, 'Third Way' politics seems to use the term 'social inclusion' to mean a focus on socially including all people in a community as a whole. 'Social inclusion' envisages an inclusive community or society for all, where partnerships, participation and shared community lead to solidarity between groups and social cohesion, which, in turn, assists in redressing social inequality. This view assumes that such an inclusive community can exist and can assert the value of solidarity, for example, while not excluding those groups whose behaviours and attitudes challenge this very solidarity. SRV theory, for example Wolfensberger (1992a, 1998), rejects this possibility and the dream of an inclusive society since one has never existed, and since all societies in order to function must reward 'in' groups, who support dominant social values and norms, and deny privileges to 'out' groups, whose characteristics, behaviours or attitudes challenge these values and norms. Without an SRV-based understanding of devaluation processes, approaches for all people effectively prioritise the needs of the more valued over the less valued and entrench devaluation as a result. Social inclusion then becomes open to abuse and can mean just about anything for devalued people, including encouraging its direct opposite, social exclusion, as the example that follows shortly shows. SRV theory would give qualified endorsement to only a few of the public health approaches specified by Kellehear (2005a), such as the "annual emergency services round table" discussion (Kellehear, 2005a, p 141). This endorsement must be a qualified one because, while a few of the programmes as described may not be explicitly devaluing, some possibility that they will not worsen the devaluation of loss and death can only exist if a raft of contextual elements entailed in the programmes also meet the requirements of SRV theory. A number of Kellehear's (2005a) other approaches are directly devaluing and create numerous new ways to further devalue people who are dying, ageing or experiencing loss and grief.

The clearest example is the "Walk-a-mile-with-me Week" (Kellehear, 2005a, p 144), where a special week is set aside every year "to assist people to understand the joys and burdens of care" through "local service or sporting clubs" visiting aged care facilities and "assisting staff in caring for the elderly for one week". The severe devaluation of such a programme appears to be unrecognised. Residents in aged care facilities are so devalued that currently they are seen as only deserving of staff with basic qualifications, yet the programme recommends that unqualified sportspeople, for example, assist in the care of such very vulnerable and mostly frail people. Besides the direct danger to life, the most transparent devaluation involved here is that the benefit of the programme accrues entirely to the carers, the institution and the valued sportspeople, while all the harm and risk is *imposed* on the devalued people. The almost total impoverishment of experience in institutional care means devalued people may enjoy out of all proportion even highly demeaning simulations of real life enjoyments that are provided in institutional care. Contrarily, such meagre enjoyment is then used as unequivocal proof of the enormous benefit to devalued people of institutional programmes. Such artificial service adaptations are institutionalised substitutions for valued or inclusive living patterns and, therefore, present numerous new opportunities to harm or otherwise further devalue vulnerable people. The unarguable goodness of the aims of such programmes masks the deep devaluation and harm involved, as Chapter Five explains in more depth. The

'Walk-a-mile-with-me Week' cannot avoid supporting the perceived rectitude of the social exclusion of older people through their institutionalisation while, at the same time, understanding itself to be promoting 'inclusive' communities. It is not only ineffectual but counterproductive to try to inspire an appreciation of the joys of caring when the mere existence of aged care institutions constructs caring for older people as an intolerable burden, at least 'eventually', and constructs ageing as a dire and frightening condition, as Chapter Five explains.

While Kellehear (2005a) acknowledges the importance of rethinking policies of institutionalisation for older people and people who are dying and addressing devalued roles, he apparently discerns a lack of power in valued roles and integration to achieve attitudinal change toward compassion. Although the intellectual disability services sector has a long way to go to address devaluation and enable people with a disability to occupy valued roles, dramatic shifts in social awareness about disability argue against Kellehear's assertion, especially when this change is measured against the systemic, inhuman treatment of not so long ago. In contrast, the central power operating in public health approaches is education. Kellehear (2005a, p 148) reminds that "compassion is more than action in time of need – it must include prevention and early intervention, and this places education at the centre of any social response". SRV theory argues that discursive means are virtually ineffectual at addressing social devaluation. A devalued person's occupancy of a valued role possesses a multidimensional power of a qualitatively different order than merely rational means because a valued role generates of itself a multitude of almost subliminal positive expectations about the role occupant.

However, Kellehear's (2005a, p 34; original emphasis) key criticism is that normalisation (or SRV) focuses on abnormality and is "*rehabilitation for some*", whereas public health approaches "enhance *the health and well-being of all*". This 'some' appears to refer to people who are dying (or devalued) as opposed to 'all' people, that is, valued people as well as devalued people. He goes on to say that "a public health approach to end-of-life care ... [understands and addresses] the *universal and normative* experiences of death, loss and grief" (Kellehear, 2005a, p 34; original emphasis). It seems he is saying that SRV can neither understand nor address the universal and normative experiences of death, loss and grief because, in his view, SRV only addresses abnormality, that is, non-normative experiences of death, loss and grief, for example, death, loss and grief related to disability. There are several major problems with this analysis, one overarching problem having already been illustrated by the case of the 'Walk-a-mile-with-me Week' programme. Any benefits of public health programmes necessarily do *not* go to 'all', but to many, the valued majority of people. And all the harm is done to the few, the 'some', the minority of devalued, vulnerable people. In the 'Walk-a-mile-with-me Week' programme, the glaring and grave risks, if only from a physical safety point of view, of sportspeople assisting with the care of frail and vulnerable residents in an aged care facility should preclude any possibility of suggesting such programmes.

There are five additional difficulties with Kellehear's (2005a) analysis. First, the inescapable reality of devaluation and the unconsciousness of devaluation, as in the 'Walk-a-mile-with-me Week' example, demand that the critical element in any approach must be to identify and focus on devaluation as devaluation, and to unilaterally and exclusively focus on compensating for this devaluation, through applying SRV principles. Protecting vulnerable people from harm has an importance of an entirely different order to any significance thought to be attached to assisting valued people with developing compassion, or educating them about the universality of loss or the 'burdens and joys of caring', no matter how beneficial such outcomes might seem for 'the community' as some kind of illusory 'all people'.

Second, when the whole social machinery is perpetuating and socialising the devaluation of people who are dying or ageing, via institutionalisation for example, the resocialising power of a compassionate book club, poster campaign, writing competition or trivial pursuit night, suggested by Kellehear (2005a), seems questionable. In any case, the unconscious devaluation that is either intrinsically embedded into these approaches, or likely to be embedded by unconscious devaluation in their contextual particularities, defeats the beneficial purpose that may be believed to exist for valued people, or 'all people'. If such approaches increase the devaluation of devalued people, then doing harm is, in fact, fostered since it is disguised as being compassionate. While being designed to create more compassionate or inclusive communities, such approaches tend to be creating communities that are actually more toxic for devalued people. The programmes mentioned convey the message that death, grief and loss, and people experiencing them, are of little consequence, the stuff of games, billboards, chitchat and competitions.

Third, Kellehear (2005a, p 34) asserts that "end-of-life care is not fully addressed by debating place of death, site of service or the integration of ageing and dying people in the community". Kellehear (2005a) appears to mean that end-of-life care involves a spectrum of broad social dimensions beyond what he sees as the restricted domains addressed by responses to devaluation and abnormality. Undoubtedly there are broader social dimensions to end-of-life care that can help valued people, or people in general, appreciate and understand loss, ageing and death. However, for devalued people, who are being subjected to relentless and inescapable devaluation, especially in an institution, these dimensions are virtually irrelevant. To repeat, it is vastly more important to stop harm being done to devalued people than it is to try to achieve any sort of generalised positive benefit for people in general.

Kellehear (2005a) seems to ignore the fact that, as Wolfensberger (2002) states, SRV is a tool that describes how to increase the valuation or devaluation of whatever social characteristic or group it is that we wish to value or devalue. If loss or end-of-life care is the characteristic whose value we want to increase, then SRV shows how to do so. To increase the value of loss, for example, there is, at some point, some relevance to maintaining/enhancing the valued social roles of valued people threatened with a diminution of status due to a loss. However, SRV theory prioritises addressing threats to people currently highly devalued by loss because the existing valued roles of valued people readily absorb, to varying degrees, threats to their status. For devalued people, on the other hand, the paucity or absence of valued roles and the plethora of their devalued roles intensify daily their lack of status. Until people who are already highly devalued because of loss are, at least, physically and to some extent socially integrated into society, any effort to address loss for 'all people' or valued people must deepen the devaluation of people already devalued by loss, if only because some attention is diverted away from the harm being done to them every day.

Public health campaigns should, therefore, first focus exclusively on devaluation, for example, via campaigns to alert all people to the toxicity of institutional care for devalued people. If devalued people are institutionalised, as in the case of older people, then there can be no groundswell of need to drive public health approaches addressing broader, less devalued social dimensions. In this case, devalued people are dependent on the goodwill of a caring society to promote and sustain public health or other approaches. This dependence is not just inappropriate but highly untrustworthy since, for devalued people, a supposedly caring society can very rapidly become a cruel society. In fact, since social processes are currently uncaring and often cruel toward devalued people, even the implication that devalued people should trust, even to a small degree, in the compassion of others invalidates the truth of the everyday experience of devalued people and, therefore, of itself devalues them.

If broader social dimensions are given a priority, then these efforts divert energy and resources away from the most devalued people and their urgent needs, and implicitly profess the rectitude of devaluation such as that occurring in institutional care. Kellehear (2005a, p 112) contends that both broader social dimensions and devaluation dimensions can, and indeed must, be addressed in tandem. SRV theory, on the contrary, stresses that all other means besides the physical and social integration of devalued people and their occupancy of valued roles are ineffectual at remediating their social devaluation. Indeed SRV theory stresses that, without physical and social integration *as a precondition* for applying any other approaches, such approaches must perpetuate and deepen existing social devaluation.

The SRV-based argument that all people, valued people as well as devalued people, are changed in the very ways Kellehear (2005a) seeks through devalued people occupying valued roles, argues against any limited effectiveness of SRV-based approaches. The evidence from the various rights movements, such as the women's movement, demonstrates the effectiveness of SRV-based outcomes. Just the presence of women in highly valued, male-dominated social roles causes a shift in what is imaginable for *every* woman, and a shift in the social value and expectancy placed on *every* woman. These valued roles have no need to educate or advocate for an empathic recognition of the commonality of the equal humanity in men and women. These valued roles prove and assert that equality and commonality directly, indisputably, with the full force of women's presence and the socially approved power accorded to these roles. The positive imagery and competency such valued roles assume and project also directly attest to the equality of women. It seems almost unimaginable that women could have attained this new valuation, and the corresponding attitudinal shifts in society, without women having become more fully integrated into valued roles in society as a precondition and proof of this revaluation. On the other hand, educational and direct attitudinal change efforts have been the approaches most readily able to be used to confirm and perpetuate devaluing stereotypes about women. These issues are pursued a little further in Chapter Seven in a brief discussion of 'identity politics' that assists in distinguishing SRV from rights-based approaches while validating the prioritising of SRV-based (and difference-based) approaches above all other means.

Fourth, communities are a central source of devaluation, divisiveness and intolerance as well as a source of solidarity, partnership and compassion. Without an SRV-based underpinning, the use of community partnerships, for example, where community members act "towards each other in new and constructive ways to improve their *own* capacity for end-of-life care" (Kellehear, 2005a, p 100; original emphasis) will almost certainly reproduce dominant devaluing tendencies toward older people or people who are dying, no matter how constructive these partnerships might seem.

Fifth, Kellehear's (2005a) fundamental criticism seems improperly constructed. The "rehabilitation for some" claim (Kellehear, 2005a, p 34) asserts that a public health approach can understand and address normative and universal loss whereas approaches specifically addressing abnormality cannot. He appears to mean that a public health approach can address all loss, loss as a universal experience, whereas approaches that address abnormal or non-normative losses, experienced by only some people, cannot. Before examining this claim, in the following discussion loss and death are used interchangeably for the sake of brevity since all loss can, to some degree, be understood as a symbol or prefiguration of death, which is consonant with Kellehear's meaning. When loss is said so is death, and vice versa.

When Kellehear (2005a, p 34; original emphasis) says "a public health approach to end-of-life care ... [understands and addresses] the *universal and normative* experiences of death, loss and grief", the meaning of the term 'normative' is not clear. The term 'normative' can be used in two ways. First, it can be used to mean statistically normative, falling within statistical frequency norms. In this sense, normative simply means numerically common, expected or likely. Second, the term 'normative' can be used to mean socially normative, included or approved by social norms and dominant values. Loss, in itself, is an abstract concept that has no practical meaning divorced from its social context. However, as soon as loss is understood as a social phenomenon, necessarily occurring in interaction with its social context, then loss is inseparable from its social normativity or non-normativity. Loss in itself or loss as-it-is, that is, as a universal and statistically normative phenomenon, has no practical social meaning.

Universal and statistically normative phenomena can be socially abnormal, non-normative or devalued, as has been discussed earlier concerning ageing, which is universal yet devalued by modern society. The present book asserts that death and dying, although universal and common experiences, are also devalued. The same applies for loss. To illustrate this devaluation with respect to loss specifically, the social norms of rampant materialistic acquisition and individualism exclude almost all relevance of loss to our lives. Loss is socially non-normative, or a social abnormality, while, at the same time, being universal and statistically normative. Kellehear (2005a, p 162) clearly asserts this fact in acknowledging that, while death and loss are both universal and normative experiences, "[t]he violence and finality of death is an affront to everything we value ...". In his view loss is, therefore, socially non-normative, abnormal or devalued, as well as statistically normative. And furthermore it is this very devaluation or marginal relevance of loss to our lives that Kellehear (2005a) wishes to address by public health measures. Contrary to the modern devaluation of loss, Kellehear (2005a) seeks to create some shift in social norms so that they become more inclusive of loss because, in his view, loss is instructive and constructive, both individually and socially. He appears to argue either that there are socially normative and socially non-normative losses, or that the statistical normativity of loss is able to deny, circumvent or transcend the social construction of loss as a socially non-normative experience. Kellehear (2005a) seems either to argue against his own stance that death, and so loss, are 'an affront to everything we value', or to confound statistical and social normativity. The statistical normativity and universality of loss cannot cause the socially embedded construction of loss as a social abnormality to be somehow made to disappear or bracketed out of consideration.

In any case, SRV theory considers the risk of social devaluation or social abnormality as a universal social phenomenon, which incidentally is also statistically normative and universal since everyone has some sort of characteristic liable to be devalued by someone. SRV theory, therefore, seeks to address the very same social abnormality of loss as public health approaches, except that SRV theory does so with greater generality since loss is merely one example of a socially devalued characteristic. Kellehear's (2005a) approaches seek to address the social abnormality of all loss. Since SRV addresses all social abnormality, which to repeat necessarily includes all loss as one example, Kellehear's (2005) assertion of a greater reach for public health approaches to loss seems problematic. Any limitation believed to apply to SRV-based approaches due to their focus on social abnormality must also apply to public health approaches to loss, since their focus is also on social abnormality in the form of loss. SRV theory can be applied to socially valued characteristics, as well as to socially devalued characteristics, and to the broader dimensions that Kellehear's (2005a) approach seeks to address, as has been said. However, SRV-based approaches choose not to focus directly on broader, less devalued dimensions because of their ineffectiveness in addressing social devaluation and their necessarily counterproductive impact while segregated environments and devalued roles dominate the landscape for a devalued class. The SRV-based analysis of the 'Walk-a-mile-with-me Week' programme demonstrates these points.

Kellehear's 'value-loss-as-it-is' version of the 'value-people-as-they-are' argument seems to say that instead of looking at loss as socially non-normative, we can step outside a "discourse of difference" (Kellehear, 2005a, p 112, citing Anthias and Yuval-Davis, 1992) into an all inclusive public health discourse by focusing on the commonality and universality of loss. Sounds good, but as has been said, the fact of the social devaluation of loss or other devalued characteristic cannot be made to disappear by shifting to a discourse that obfuscates this fact, or by pretending that it is a false or illusory social imposition, attribution or construction. The following illustration briefly explores how this construction of devaluation is almost subliminally embedded into social context.

Kellehear (2005a, p 140) suggests conducting 'trivial pursuit nights' with, for example, a focus on raising awareness about the commonality of loss. SRV theory explains, as SRV core themes described later in this chapter show, that embedded devaluing social imagery pervades the social context of devalued characteristics. SRV theory explains that such nights would convey the messages that death and loss are trivial; that they can be fun and fun for all; that they are a game; that if we all eat, drink and be merry together we can all understand loss and death as a commonality; that death and loss pursue us; that death's pursuit of humanity is trivial; that death and loss are connected with night and darkness and so on. There are also many cultural overlays that devalue a variety of groups from trivial pursuit's origins as a Canadian/US game for the idle affluent. And this is not taking into account another vast array of devaluing imagery that is bound to be embedded into the particular context in which such trivial pursuit nights would be held, such as the title of the night, the groups who attend, the people who sponsor and organise, the people who donate prizes, the type of prizes, the setting, the location, the subject matter, the questions/answers, the reading information distributed, the manner of distribution, the advertising flyers, the location of flyers and so on. Since the social devaluation of loss is mediated by social norms, every context in which loss is raised is pervaded by a vast array of devaluation processes, both actual and potential.

Chapter Seven explores in a little more detail these issues around the idea that a public health approach or other discourse that does not exclusively focus on difference decontextualises loss, death and devalued difference, in general. Loss and death are not problems in themselves. The social devaluation of loss and death is the problem, because this devaluation marginalises the relevance of loss and death to our lives. All thinking about social devaluation or difference, especially thinking that tries to look beyond devalued difference, as if not naming it as difference could deny its devaluation, needs to clearly distinguish between the devalued characteristic itself and the devaluation attending the devalued characteristic. This fundamental distinction is vital in order to understand how devaluation operates and how devaluing effects are necessarily hidden and embedded in approaches that do not focus on difference as a devalued characteristic. This distinction is used in Chapter Seven to direct a reconceptualisation of death that further clarifies Kellehear's (2005a) universalisation of loss and death.

Ten core themes of SRV

Role of (un)consciousness (Wolfensberger, 1998, p 103)

"No one is exempt from becoming entrapped into unconsciousness ... [of, for example,] the reality, extent, and dynamics of social devaluation,... the transmission of image messages,... and the real functions of many human services" (Wolfensberger, 1998, pp 103-4). SRV aims to make conscious the unconscious processes of devaluation (and valuation) (Wolfensberger, 1998, p 104). This process has also been termed 'conscientisation' by Friere (1972) or consciousness-raising, as noted by Race (1999, p 108).

The following are examples of the relevance of this theme to palliative care:

- Significant, unrecognised, harmful effects of palliative care must exist.
- Individuals, organisations and society as a whole will be, to some degree, unconscious of the processes of devaluation concerning people who are dying.
- The goodness of palliative care and its religious ethos tends to hide the mechanisms of devaluation by the palliative care system and its practitioners.

In their development of a five-part model for the eradication of the 'dark side of nursing' (Jameton, 1992), that is, the stigmatising and harmful side, Corley and Goren (1998) specify two requirements to address unconsciousness in nursing. These are first, to acknowledge the reality of the 'dark side' and second, to "develop an ethically conscious culture" (Corley and Goren, 1998, p 110). With nursing's central role in palliative care, these directives toward the eradication of unconsciousness assume a critical importance. SRV theory explains ways by which such admonitions can be put into practice.

Dynamics and relevance of social imagery (Wolfensberger, 1998, p 104)

Paraphrasing Wolfensberger (1998, p 104), image association is extremely powerful as is shown in psychology, education and advertising, for example. Even unconscious image messages are extremely powerful, and are especially so due to their penetration of conscious mental filters. "The symbols and imagery that have historically been associated with devalued people relentlessly represent negatively valued elements and qualities: animality, illness,…" and the rest of the elements of the stereotypical devalued roles (Wolfensberger, 1998, p 104). The aim is to convey positive, but realistic, image messages about devalued people.

The following are examples of the relevance of this theme to palliative care:

- The cultural analogues to group dying are war, famine, contagion or genocide. Therefore, these kinds of images and their impacts are evoked by collecting together a group of people to die in palliative care institutions.
- The images attending medical and religious organisations and personnel are transposed into palliative care.
- Situating a palliative care service in/near a hospital conveys the images of sickness, treatment and cure; near a church conveys images associated with holiness and religion; near a funeral company conveys the image that people who are dying are already dead; in/near a kindergarten conveys that people who are dying are childlike or to be treated or understood as children; in a rural retreat-type environment conveys the image of the object of dread, to be isolated, contained and separated, only able to be managed by such grand measures.

Architectural insight into the negative messages generated by palliative care services vividly illustrates that, although palliative care ideology asserts the value of people who are dying (or dead), the actual message given by the social imagery surrounding palliative care contradicts this value position. Valins et al (1996, pp 109-10) note some hospices "where visitors enter the vicinity through a carefully planned canopy or porte-cochere, yet patients are brought in via the service entrance. The deceased leave spectacularly ungraciously via the service centre which in some cases is near the refuse bins". Such mechanisms of devaluation propagate and reflect the social image of people who are dying, or have died, as worthless commodities, only worthy of being treated like discarded rubbish, unworthy of coming and going by the same means that valued citizens come and go. This "rubbish or waste role" (Race, 1999, p 56) is a variant of the stereotypical devalued role of 'already dead'.

Power of mindsets and expectancies (Wolfensberger, 1998, p 105)

Our expectations about a person shape our perceptions of him/her, and influence the nature of our responses to him/her. SRV aims to

> ... shape the mind-sets and expectancies that people hold about various devalued persons and classes so that these mind-sets (a) are as positive as realistically possible, (b) presume the presence of potential for growth and development, (c) expect such to take place, and (d) expect people to fill valued rather than devalued roles in society. (Wolfensberger, 1998, p 105)

The following are examples of the relevance of this theme to palliative care:

- The mindsets of practitioners conform to the prescribed expectations of the medical, religio-charitable and palliative care models.
- Maintaining the role of home owner/occupier by not admitting a person to a hospice maintains or defends this crucial valued role and its competencies and positive imagery. Institutionalisation eliminates this role.

Relevance of role expectancy and role circularity to deviancy making and deviancy unmaking (Wolfensberger, 1998, p 106)

"The dynamics of role expectancy and role circularity are ever-present in human life and very familiar to just about everyone" (Wolfensberger, 1998, pp 106-7). The self-fulfilling prophecy is an example. There is a "feedback loop" (Wolfensberger, 1998, p 75) between a person's role and the set of expectancies this role conveys. Valued roles lead to positive expectations, which lead to more-valued roles, which lead to more positive expectations and so on. And there is a similar feedback loop between devalued roles and negative expectations. The feedback loop for a valued role implies that positive expectations lead to increasingly valued status and, for a devalued role that negative expectations lead to increasingly devalued status. By manipulating these feedback processes, deviancy or devalued status can be made or unmade (Wolfensberger, 1998).

The following are examples of the relevance of this theme to palliative care:

- The messages conveyed by the ideology, structure, settings and service user roles likely to be prescribed in palliative care form what people expect of people who are dying. These expectations become what we observe in people who are dying, just as specific stage theory behaviours, such as denial, were falsely observed.
- Behaviours, attitudes and symptoms of all sorts may be caused, suppressed or exacerbated by the effects of social devaluation.
- The messages conveyed by wide-ranging religio-charitable connotations cause people who are dying and the services who care for them to be perceived as special, that is, romantically idealised.

Personal competency enhancement and the developmental model (Wolfensberger, 1998, p 108)

The developmental model considers that "all people have the potential for positive responsiveness at all stages in their lives, no matter how old or impaired they are; that there exists a vast array of means to help people move closer to actualizing their potential" (Wolfensberger, 1998, p 109). People's often unconscious assumptions can reflect different beliefs to the developmental model.

Different professionals can often hold mutually contradictory assumptions about cause and effect. Medicine tends to see biological illness, and then treatment through drugs. Psychologists tend to see emotional or psychological issues, and their resolution through dialogue and self-reflective work. The developmental model circumvents such operative assumptions by stressing that every behaviour entails competencies that should be the focus of enhancement or preservation. This is not to say that problems should be disregarded and competencies become the sole focus, but rather that emphasis on the problem and its treatment, under whatever assumptions, can mean that the competencies exhibited in the problem are not recognised, not valued and allowed to wither. In palliative care, repeated angry behaviour may cause the suspicion of cerebral metastatic disease or grieving troubles, family problems or anger at God and the relevant remedy pursued, while competencies inherent in the behaviour such as communication, courage, self-advocacy or assertiveness and direct physical competencies may not be identified specifically and preserved. Again, this is not to say that the possible issues causing such behaviour should be ignored, especially justifiable reasons for expressing anger, but that, at least, the person exhibiting angry behaviour should be understood as always communicating something, and be made aware of competencies or strengths in the behaviour and their value, both actual and potential. The developmental model considers the effect of every contextual element, such as the surroundings, the process and staff expertise, in order to utilise contexts that promote the maximum development of competencies (Wolfensberger, 1998).

The following are examples of the relevance of this theme to palliative care:

- Each team discipline brings its model's assumptions, which may contradict each other and the developmental model on which palliative care is based.
- The entire context of palliative care, not just its programmes, should be examined to determine the extent to which a context facilitates competency enhancement and growth. A programme or philosophy of care cannot be separated from the context in which it is delivered.
- Practitioners with significant expertise in an area will best develop a person's competencies in that area.

Concepts of relevance, potency, and model coherency of measures and services (Wolfensberger, 1998, p 111)

Wolfensberger (1998, pp 108-10) considers a human service as exhibiting coherence/incoherence between its assumptions, contents and processes. "Relevance means that the content addresses a major or significant need" of service users and, therefore, that the "most urgent" needs are addressed first (Wolfensberger, 1998, p 111). Potency refers to using the most "effective and efficient" processes (Wolfensberger, 1998, p 113).

Together relevance and potency make up the idea of 'model coherency'. Many flaws in common service models derive from poor model coherency, for example, by applying the medical model to people who are dying – an acute to a chronic care context – since medical needs, once relatively stable, are not the most urgent need for the vast majority of people who are dying. A primary problem in model coherency arises from using processes that create new needs or increase existing needs (Wolfensberger, 1998, p 117). For example, the definitional inclusion of nursing or pastoral care in the palliative care interdisciplinary team images death and dying as medical and religious/ spiritual processes requiring, at least potentially, the services of such disciplines. The point is not that palliative care may not or should not include nursing or spiritual needs, far from it, but that the current service model that defines the interdisciplinary team in this way conveys a whole range of ideas about death and dying that can create further problems for people who are dying. The current definition of a palliative care team assumes each person could, should or does need nursing/ medical care, social, pastoral and psychological support and the involvement of volunteers, or some elements thereof.

With palliative care portrayed in this way, the community comes to define its needs regarding death and dying within these same parameters. For this kind of reason, the cultural and disease selectiveness of palliative care may indicate the inappropriateness of this definition to non-dominant cultural or disease groups. If a model "does not make sense to members of a culture", then this is one key sign of model incoherency (Wolfensberger, 1998, p 117). In palliative care, the lack of utilisation of hospice care by people with diseases other than cancer, or by minority cultural groups, points to the model's incoherency.

Model coherency is an important idea for understanding SRV. In studying model coherency the most powerful tool to reveal how to adjust the structure of systems to be more socially valuing is known as the "culturally valued analogue" (Wolfensberger, 1998, p 118), as discussed by Race (1999, pp 136-9). The coherence of any service aspect with respect to its assumptions, contents and processes can be examined by considering the question: how would a person highly valued by the dominant culture routinely want or have this need addressed, or routinely want or have this service provided? The pattern of care that is the answer to this question then becomes the 'culturally valued analogue' against which patterns of care for devalued people can be compared. The model coherency is high if the service aspect approximates very closely to the culturally valued analogue.

Analysis of the basic approaches of palliative care services using the culturally valued analogue reveals a high level of incoherency. Would a wealthy businessman routinely choose a hospice or hospital as the place in which to die? Would a doctor routinely choose a volunteer to provide, for example, counselling, meditation services or companionship? Would a professor or bishop routinely choose the local palliative day care centre or palliative care agency to provide massage, craft or social interaction? Would a lawyer routinely choose a nurse to deliver holistic aspects of care, such as counselling or spiritual care? Not only does the culturally valued analogue expose hidden, that is, unconscious ways in which services devalue people, but it also points to ways to adjust service elements so that they become more valuing.

The following are examples of the relevance of this theme for palliative care:

- Parameters for services' structures and processes should be set by comparison with the culturally valued analogues relating to each element in service provision.
- Institutional care creates a whole new set of problems, such as travelling problems for the carer, as a minor illustration, or loss of home for the person who is dying, as a crucial illustration.

Importance of interpersonal identification between valued and devalued people (Wolfensberger, 1998, p 118)

When a valued and devalued person identify with each other, the valued person is more likely to seek and enable positive outcomes for the devalued person, who is likely to model him/herself on the behaviour and competencies of the valued person (Wolfensberger, 1998, p 119). Interpersonal identification between valued and devalued people is an "intermediate goal" toward valued social roles (Wolfensberger, 1998, p 120).

The following are examples of the relevance of this theme to palliative care:

- Participating in their own community allows people who are dying to retain their valued social roles and allows interpersonal identification between people who are dying and members of their community.
- Relationships with valued people (who are not staff of services) via interpersonal identification offer the greatest safeguard against abuse, negligence, the denial of rights, and poor service quality.
- The diversity of the ordinary community allows people who are dying to maintain a mix of valued interactions and not be restricted to socially devalued interactions with the therapeutic community or with other service users.

Pedagogic power of imitation, via modelling and interpersonal identification (Wolfensberger, 1998, p 120)

> Devalued persons are commonly (a) segregated away from valued society and models, (b) congregated with (other) devalued people who ... exhibit socially devalued behaviours, and (c) served by less competent workers than typically serve valued people. (Wolfensberger, 1998, p 120)

The following are examples of the relevance of this theme to palliative care:

- From nursing care to interpersonal behaviour to organisational information, modelling inculcates the prescribed culture of palliative care.
- When people who are dying are congregated together they will imitate other recipients of care and the therapeutic community of the setting.
- The use of voluntary labour is devaluing since no valued organisation such as a global corporation, or valued person such as a lawyer, would routinely use voluntary labour in providing their direct services.

Importance of personal social integration and valued social participation especially for people at risk of social devaluation (Wolfensberger, 1998, p 122)

> [D]evalued people who are segregated are thereby denied normative, typical experiences that valued members of society take for granted, ... [segregation of a devalued group] may reduce the society's level of tolerance for diversity (Wolfensberger, 1998, p 122).

> 'Integration' ... [requires] (a) valued participation, (b) with valued people (c) in valued activities that (d) take place in valued settings (Wolfensberger, 1998, p 123).

The following are examples of the relevance of this theme to palliative care:

- All segregated environments such as hospices, inpatient palliative care units, nursing homes, hospice houses and day care centres are devaluing and inappropriate.
- Organisations that deny or reduce inclusion by providing the majority of services themselves or by duplicating services already available in the community, such as generic nursing or medical services, hairdressing or complementary therapy services, are devaluing and inappropriate.

'Conservatism corollary,' or the concept of positive compensation for devalued status (Wolfensberger, 1998, p 124)

"[Devalued] people ... or [people] who are at risk of such devaluation are much more vulnerable to being further devalued ... as a result of even minor devalued characteristics" (Wolfensberger, 1998, p 124). Compensating for devalued status involves reducing the number of vulnerabilities of a person/group, and/or reducing the size of any group of devalued people, and/or increasing associations with valued people, characteristics, settings and so on (Wolfensberger, 1998, p 126). Where there is a choice between a moderately valued and a highly valued option for a devalued person, the more highly valued option better protects against devaluation.

The following are examples of the relevance of this theme to palliative care:

- One devalued characteristic is unremarkable. When this characteristic is multiplied by grouping people who are dying together, the intensified visibility multiplies the devaluation and encourages the 'freak show' mentality.
- Using quality offices, materials, settings, venues, vehicles, staff, equipment and so on protects against social devaluation.

FIVE

Implications for palliative care

Introduction

Rather than analysing the palliative care system by exploring the specific implications of each core theme, the implications of four key principles that bring together essential SRV ideas and core themes are discussed. These four principles or objectives define the kinds of approaches that SRV requires of service systems. The significance of these principles for palliative care approaches is examined under each principle. All four principles have implications concerning institutionalisation because the institution of care is the clearest and most extreme example of how a service system establishes and perpetuates social devaluation. The inherent effects of institutions are discussed separately because the impact of institutional expression is so widely misunderstood and so prevalent in health care systems, especially palliative care. It is argued that analysing the palliative care system using these SRV-based principles demonstrates significant and widespread social devaluation throughout the palliative care system.

The mindset of the 'benevolent institution myth' (Harris, 1995) believes that the institutional model is both necessary and benevolent. However, SRV theory argues that in all non-acute contexts of care the institutional model is neither necessary nor benevolent, especially for people at risk of social devaluation. The reasons people choose institutional care are the same irrespective of the particular context of care, and reflect people's inherited beliefs about institutional models rather than the empirical realities of institutional life.

After exploring four key SRV-based principles, this chapter discusses the 'benevolent institution myth', including the reasons used to justify institutional care. Seven inescapable paradoxes of institutional models that undermine the claims of the 'benevolent institution myth' are then described with reference to the palliative care context.

Applying SRV to palliative care

Identify unconscious devaluation from imported models

Palliative care has imported aspects of the medical, religio-charitable and medico-psychological models of care, as well as having imported the professionalised model of modern human service delivery. Identifying the ways these models express themselves in palliative care assists in identifying devaluing mechanisms imported into palliative care.

"The hospice movement at least in North America ... comes to us largely as a faddish and perverted variation of a meritorious old theme, and its actual as well as potentially dangerous elements are virtually unrecognised and unacknowledged by most of the many people who enthusiastically embrace it" (Wolfensberger, 1984, p 167). Wolfensberger's overriding concern in this quote is the general issue that a legitimisation of a virtual eradication of devalued groups, such as people with a chronic condition or disability, might be established via the hospice movement. Nevertheless, his statement underlines his perception of the extent of the unconsciousness of the harm able to be caused by social devaluation in the (US) hospice movement.

Palliative care's high social approval tends to discourage criticism and encourage the presumption that harm is not being done. Teamwork in palliative care illustrates this point. Although, as Robbins (1998, p 91) points out, the belief in the effectiveness of the team philosophy in palliative care is fundamental, little research has been undertaken in this area. While effective teamwork of interdisciplinary palliative care teams is frequently asserted (for example, Parry, 1989; West, 1990), such claims may instead reflect the power of palliative care's culture to ensure conformity among its members. Zollo (1999, p 26) connects Barr's (1993) 'groupthink', where actual teamwork is nominal since no disagreement occurs, with Street's (1995, p 30) "tyranny of niceness" in nursing culture, where nurses put aside their feelings so as to not make a fuss. Within palliative care culture, this 'niceness' exists very strongly since it comes with the models imported into palliative care. The religious roots of nursing and care in general, the stereotypical role of women in nursing, professional caring and society, and the ethos of religious foundations and charitable organisations, all predispose palliative care to a culture of 'niceness'. The expectation, from the 'tyranny of niceness' and palliative care culture in general, to repress criticism entrenches palliative care's unconsciousness of its harmful effects as a system of care.

From an SRV-based perspective, being unconscious of devaluation means that harm is being done not only, as Saunders (1977) identifies, as a result of accidental flaws in interpersonal relating or the work of individual practitioners but, as a result of the very structures and processes of palliative care. Unconsciousness of the nature of devaluation allows any model of care to claim benevolence and propagate this myth that harm is only done by careless or accidental mistakes by individual practitioners, rather than identifying the ways harm is structured into the way care is organised and provided. Palliative care itself came into being, in part, to reform the whole approach of the dominant institutional medical services for people who were dying. The fault did not simply lie with individual practitioners in the hospitalised care of people who were dying. These practitioners were one small element in a whole system and culture that caused harm and needed to be changed. As a result, hospice care aimed to be an entirely different culture, a whole new way of caring and organising care, because the old way did harm, for the most part unconsciously. A new system needed to be created with different definitions, goals, structures and processes as well as different individual attitudes.

McKnight (1995) draws attention to the underlying agenda of all human service systems. He considers that the human service system serves vested interests that are not those of the people who need support. "The enemy is not poverty, sickness and disease", and dying/death could be added to this list. "The enemy is a set of institutions and interests that are advantaged by clienthood and dependency" which is "masked by service" (McKnight, 1995, pp 98-9). McKnight's (1995, p 99) 'wanted list' of enemies in this regard powerfully evokes the enormous degree of the denial of citizenship rights resulting from self-serving institutional interests. Palliative care's institutional interests and their unconscious influence on the way care is provided are a part of this broader impact.

Model incoherence is a key way devaluing tendencies come about and remain hidden. Incoherence frequently arises from contradictions between palliative care assumptions and those of the models imported into palliative care. For example, the holistic interdisciplinary palliative care team is a direct transposition to the palliative care context of the hierarchical multidisciplinary team of the hospital. However, since assumptions about community in the religious ethos override, in palliative care, the assumptions of the medical model concerning the effectiveness of a hierarchical structure for decision making, the hierarchical hospital team has to become a non-hierarchical team in palliative care, at least conceptually. Despite its implausibility it is asserted, as Zollo (1999, p 30) indicates, that the therapeutic community or team of the palliative care unit has managed, by means such as team "education and open communication", to overcome team status differentials that obtain within society or the medical framework at large. Palliative care assumes that a non-hierarchical team or community can be developed while retaining the fundamental hierarchical team structure and composition of the acute setting. This type of incoherence allows devaluation to be imported unconsciously from the hospital model.

The term 'medical model', a central element of the paradigm of care, refers to the whole construction of modern medicine, some of which has been outlined in various respects in Chapter Two, chiefly under the first key feature, institutional expression and role system. The term is now used to refer primarily to the hospital model and its influence. Importing aspects of the acute care medical model to a chronic care context, such as palliative care, must introduce significant incoherence. Just as the hospital was carried over into palliative care as the hospice, so too was the organisation of the hospital. For example, the process of referral from key ward staff (nurses/doctors) to a specific set of ancillary disciplines is replicated within the palliative care team. Palliative care uses mostly medical structures, processes, language and symbols because the medical model dominates palliative care. So there are ward, nursing station, patient, patient history, diagnosis, prognosis, symptom management, progress notes, clinical care, nursing rosters/ shifts, handover and so on. Palliative care, via its medical expression, cannot avoid carrying over role and status differentials operative within the medical system, such as those between consultant and GP, as well as medical imperatives such as the demand to conduct research and teaching in an institution.

Palliative care terminology is not coherent across its constituent disciplines. Other contexts are overlaid onto the medical. Therefore, there are also: clients, not patients; files, not records; assessments or listening to a person's story, not diagnosis; case notes, not progress notes; problems, issues, concerns, spiritual challenges or opportunities for growth, not symptoms; intervention, 'working through' or 'working with', not treatment; and so on. The composition of direct care personnel in palliative care is the same as the hospital: doctor, nurse, social worker, pastoral carer/chaplain and volunteer with some allied health component (for example, massage, physiotherapy or complementary therapies) available when extra expertise is thought to be required by nursing/medical staff. The interdisciplinary palliative care team and its processes are a direct transposition from the hospital ward, even though this transposition is overlaid with nuances from other contexts and models.

Clark and Seymour's (1999, p 87, pp 112-24) discussion of "important etymological and definitional problems" reveals the lack of clarity about what hospice care is, as well as confusion about the nature of medicalisation and 'routinisation' (James and Field, 1992). For example Salisbury (1997, p 48), referred to by Clark and Seymour (1999, p 166), can maintain that "the philosophy of hospice ... involves a personal, non-institutional approach" when the founding principles are those of a religio-medical type of care developed within an institution and, for the most part, centred on an institution. As discussed in Chapter Three, Saunders' conceptualisation is explicitly medical (therefore, it cannot be demedicalised), is explicitly religious (therefore, it cannot be non-religious), and is explicitly institutional (therefore, it cannot be non-institutional). Religio-medicalised, institutional approaches must, therefore, pervade modern palliative care whether it is delivered in an institution or in a private home by a community-based or hospice-based palliative care service. Influential institutional approaches can be overcome only by changing the whole construction and organisation of palliative care. It seems obvious that such potent systemic influences cannot be overcome, or significantly ameliorated, by using some voluntary labour (deprofessionalising), or by emphasising nurses more than doctors (demedicalising), or by employing secular staff (making non-religious), or by allowing a few simple flexibilities in institutional regimes (making non-institutional). These strange service adaptations by palliative care create new incoherence, and so new ways of devaluing people who are dying.

While this sort of unacknowledged importation of the medical model remains, hidden and extensive medicalisation must follow. For example, as noted earlier, the influence of the hospital ward model situates nurses in the primary case management role that makes referrals to other members of the team. A hidden or unconscious medicalisation of holistic assessment must, therefore, take place. Nursing and its image associations, such as illness, hospital, compliance, sanitised regimented environments and maternal caring, are thereby constructed as the primary identifiers of palliative care, since nurses have colonised the primary or case management assessment function.

Despite importing incoherency from its constituent models, an integrated model commonly considers itself coherent, in other words, that it has integrated without contradiction the various constituent models and their various assumptions, contents and processes. Functional problems in the integrated model are, therefore, assumed to arise from internal processes or contents in the integrated model, when very often the root of functional problems lies in clashes between the integrated model's assumptions, processes and contents and those of its constituent models. In the example already discussed, status problems in team functioning may be thought to arise from such things as interpersonal team dynamics, whereas these apparently functional difficulties are much more likely to derive from importing hospital ward structures and processes and their associated status differentials. Using team-building exercises to improve team functioning can have little effect, if the difficulty arises from imported status differentials that still obtain in other contexts. The only solution can be to identify the structures and processes that enable this transference of status and reconfigure them.

Other key 'functional' problems that derive from importing medical assumptions include the specialist–generalist dilemma about how these different levels of expertise should work together in direct care, and also the marginalisation of the psychosocial/spiritual team, concerning both case management and direct care. These and many additional 'functional' problems, such as the ever-expanding scope and expertise requirement of palliative care nursing practice, can be resolved if an understanding develops about the ways the hospital ward model has been imported into palliative care. Problems concerning the scope of palliative care nursing practice, for example, are not due to the ever-widening needs of diverse palliative care users but rather due to the assumptions underlying the institutional medical model about who should service which needs. The hospital ward requires that all care be delivered on the ward by the ward/hospital staff. Under these assumptions, and the organisation that manifests them, it seems irresponsible to suggest that the scope of palliative care nursing practice does not have to be able to encompass the whole range of needs. In the same way it seems irresponsible to suggest that palliative care specialist expertise does not need to be rationed and reserved for 'difficult cases', which is the medical model's solution or assumption about how to integrate the two levels of expertise (generalist/specialist). In palliative care under this assumption, the problem reduces to an insoluble dilemma: "whether to provide high quality services to a few people or to provide lesser services for greater numbers?" (James and Field, 1992, p 1372).

However, before alternative assumptions can be understood, the impact of assumptions of the models underpinning palliative care must be understood. The author's experience in partially reconfiguring a specialist palliative care service along SRV-based lines indicates that a model that addresses devaluation can also resolve a whole array of these long-standing dilemmas. For example, if nurses are not structured into the primary case management role then the dislocation and loss caused to family/carers and nurses when care patterns change on bereavement, which is noted by Aranda (1993), can be significantly reduced. By addressing the underlying devaluation, incoherent processes and assumptions become more coherent and problems either vanish or moderate considerably as a result.

Social integration

A key safeguard against social devaluation comes from valued people identifying with devalued people through valued interactions in valued settings where valued people usually interact. Palliative care systems need to facilitate these interactions and eradicate segregated environments for the care of people who are dying where, necessarily, everything is abnormal.

Robbins (1998, p 102) notes that "the literature on palliative care objectives, service specifications, and standards is strong on assertion and rhetoric, but weak on the evidence to back up the claims of what palliative care staff actually do". Palliative care's "anecdotal success and emotional appeal" (Robbins, 1998, p 146, citing Lunt and Hillier, 1981), together with its sometimes sentimental rhetoric, convey an extraordinariness or specialness about palliative care, its environments and outcomes. That palliative care promotes these kinds of exceptional attributions demonstrates a key element of its unconsciousness about the way social devaluation operates. The extraordinary interactions, settings, communities and effects claimed by hospice, for example by Saunders (1977), are precisely those things that deny interpersonal identification between ordinary valued people outside the therapeutic community and people who are dying. Extraordinary structures and processes, and especially extraordinary outcomes, mystify death, dying and palliative care as extraordinary. These claims to extraordinariness work against making death, dying and palliative care 'normal' parts of living. Echoing Robbins (1998), Connor (1998, p 114) states that after 30 years: "What is striking is the lack of serious research being done in the field of palliative care in the US. Many of the studies that are published are small in scale or lack methodological sophistication". Connor (1998, p 114) refers to the "paucity of research", particularly concerning the quality of palliative care. Connor (1998, p 114) states that two questions among others "have yet to be answered, but must be addressed: 'Is hospice care better than traditional care?' and 'What are the measurable outcomes of hospice care?"'.The rhetoric, anecdotes and claims of hospice, as well as its social approval, need to be understood against this background.

Palliative care systems are a mutation of the specialist hospital system with outpatient and outreach services. Notwithstanding the dogma that palliative care is a programme or philosophy of care able to be applied in any setting, the central pillar and symbol of the palliative care system is its institution. SRV theory emphasises that segregation is an inherent, inescapable and defining function of any institution. An exacerbation of the stigma associated with the devalued class in institutional care chiefly occurs because of the negative impact of the images and practices involved in grouping devalued people together. Institutions disallow external scrutiny and their size, authority and status emasculate criticism and efforts to seek recompense for unjust, improper or negligent practice. Institutions destroy, deny, replace or restructure inmates' connections with their normal community. Portraying themselves as the repositories of ultimate expertise, institutions convey the message that alternative ways of caring are inferior and that choosing an alternative approach represents a morally irresponsible course of action.

Wolfensberger (1984, p 168) asserts that the most meritorious aspect of (US) hospice care is that it extends care into people's homes. A person's normal patterns of living and his/her valued social roles are able to be preserved if the home (as the standard role-valorising environment) is the central focus of the care system, rather than the institution. Strauss (1994) asserts that the (US) healthcare system must shift its organisational emphasis from the hospital and clinic to the home. In Strauss' (1994) view, the medical model centred on the hospital has already fallen well short of meeting the need for chronic care, particularly for devalued groups, which is and increasingly will become the main demand on the system. Palliative care models such as Maddocks' (1990, p 537) "triangle of care", which depicts three sites of care – home, hospital and hospice – as an interconnected triangle, suggest an integration of the home into the care system. However, mostly such models seem to take little account of institutional agenda and the dominant institutional model at work in the system and, therefore, simply perpetuate institutions as the centre of care.

SRV theory emphasises that communities and attitudes can only become valuing if interactions between valued and devalued people actually take place in these communities. Devalued and valued people both have the opportunity to learn how to communicate with each other that is, in palliative care, in the ordinary lived reality where one party is dying. Interactions should take place in valued settings where normal, valued pursuits take place. Institutions of care are extraordinary realities, if only because they collect people with the same sort of devalued characteristic together. Living patterns, where dying is a part of the community's experience, can only be established if people actually remain in their homes until they die there. Dying is not normalised by people living in their homes for the majority of the last year of their life, yet not in fact dying there. The ultimate deviance of death and dying is reinforced in these circumstances because dying tends to become divorced from death. Dying is redefined, reducing to a very short, 'acute' terminal phase, and palliative care is reduced to end-stage care. People who are dying, while remaining in their community in their own homes, live with the good and the bad encountered among people living in any normal community. People may experience stimulation, comfort, companionship and pleasure from others, as well as ignorance, rejection and patronisation. A therapeutic community claims it has eradicated or managed 'bad' outside influences, although actually such closed 'counterfeit' (McKnight, 1995) communities and environments create new ways for bad things to happen. The more important point here is, however, that if the 'bad' is excluded in a sanitised, protective, therapeutic environment then the 'bad' cannot be challenged and remediated in the places where it actually occurs. The community, therefore, becomes less and less able to understand the difference known as dying, and to respond to it.

Institutions where group dying occurs create an atypical visibility, which is useful for institutional purposes, such as gaining credibility and respectability, concealing the problematic condition, conducting research and generating philanthropic support. However, inappropriate or atypical visibility entrenches the social devaluation of people who are dying. Highly valued people in society would use their increased resources to avoid dying in institutional care with other people who are dying. If palliative care seeks to value people who are dying then the option that a highly valued person would choose should be the goal for all. Configuring a system around the expectation that this goal can never be reached makes this expectation become the unavoidable reality. Whether the goal for every person to have the resources he/she needs to die at home is claimed to be too idealistic or too costly, these arguments are, at bottom, statements about social priorities. The message is the same: people who are dying are not a sufficiently high priority to deserve the resources required, or to warrant a shift in ideal. The cost of supporting people to die in their homes currently does not appear to be a relevant factor in the denial of home death to the vast majority. Clark and Seymour (1999, p 158) state: "as well as being more acceptable to patients and carers, the cost of home-based palliative care is significantly less than in-patient care".

However, under an institutional model, resources can only be used to foster the institutional way, epitomised by Fisher (1996) who conveys the typical grand, therapeutic image of hospice. In response to the question "where do we start [when we want to build a hospice]?" Fisher (1996, p 83) answers: "get as big a garden as you can, and put your building in the middle of it". Such pronouncements appear to consider therapeutic propensity as the main priority in assessing the appropriateness of a service development, an approach typical of the religio-charitable and clinical perspectives.

SRV theory would assert as a self-evident truth that, no matter how therapeutic a hospice garden might be, it can never replace a person's own garden. The hospice interpretation of therapeutic is decontextualised. A person suffers the loss of his/her own garden, because palliative care adopts institutional care as a mode of care, and is then provided with a grand hospice garden therapy substitute. Ironically, this is done, in part, to help ease the loss from institutionalisation, of which the loss of garden may be one element. Resituating people who have lost their own garden in a grand, therapeutic garden is not only ironic but could very well be interpreted as an insult. However, grand and caring gestures preclude service users owning up to any such feelings, much less expressing them or criticising palliative care. The deindividualisation intrinsic to institutional approaches is also evident because, although some people hate large gardens, or any sort of garden, or may even have allergic or phobic reactions to them, in a hospice with a garden people have no choice but to have that particular hospice garden.

Social integration is more than just the physical integration, as opposed to the segregation, of the service setting. Social inclusion, that is, valued participation with valued people in valued settings, means going to the local library to read about dying rather than to the hospice library. It means attending a local meditation group with 'non-dying' people, not attending meditation run by cancer services or palliative care units. It means using one's own doctor, nurse, chaplain, hairdresser, counsellor, complementary therapist and so on as one normally accesses these services, not replacing all these services with those of the palliative care service, simply because the person is dying. It means driving through one's own neighbourhood being recognised by and recognisable to the people and the environment. It means praying with one's own religious community, not the hospice community or, alternatively, it may mean never being in an environment where people with a religious ethos congregate. It means enjoying one's own garden in the same way that a valued person might. It means supporting one's socially valued roles rather than replacing the ordinary living patterns in which one is established with imitations, no matter how beneficial or therapeutic these may seem.

Every effort to substitute for lost roles tries to mask the implied insult or mockery contained in such efforts. One's ordinary life is worthy of imitation on a grand scale, but not worthy of preservation. Very few people want to live in nursing homes, yet these continue to be built everywhere. The most socially valued among us would never live in such places. Very few people would choose to die in an institution rather than their own home, yet we keep on supporting a system in which the vast majority, except the most socially valued, will die in an institution. Continuing in this way, a system is perpetuated that denies the privileges enjoyed by the most socially valued to those less socially valued. A palliative care (and aged care) system is continuing to be constructed in which institutional agenda are placed ahead of the wishes of almost all people who are dying or ageing. The adage remains as true as ever: 'if you build an institution, it will be filled'. And the institution will be filled if only to validate the necessity and excellence of the institution.

It is not clear what Saunders (1995, p xiii) means when she says: "hospice is about living until the end, still as part of the community". She seems to use the term 'community' not to refer to the hospice user's local community of origin and his/her valued roles and place in that community, but in some much broader, or even abstract, sense. This seemingly misleading usage allows a positive spin to be put on the radical excision from one's community that is institutionalisation.

Defend valued roles

To show we value a person, we seek to enable, defend, maintain or enhance their valued roles. As a corollary, we seek to eliminate any of their devalued roles and avoid people entering new devalued roles (Wolfensberger, 1998, pp 84-95). In palliative care, our primary concerns should be to maintain people's valued roles, such as home owner/occupier, and avoid people entering a whole array of new, devalued roles upon institutionalisation.

Wolfensberger (1972, 1975, 1998) describes the stereotypical negative roles ascribed to devalued people, which have been listed in Chapter

Four. The bad things that are done to people cast into these stereotypical, devalued roles include: rejection, distancing (physically and socially), impoverishment of experience, loss of freely given relationships, "social and relationship discontinuity", discontinuity with physical objects including possessions, loss of control, deindividualisation and involuntary poverty (Wolfensberger, 1998, pp 12-24). Many of these bad things can also be found in the palliative care context. For example, Kellehear (1990, p 52, citing Simpson, 1979) describes some of the social reactions that occur to people with a terminal illness as "discrimination, sacking, intrusion, gossip, overprotection and the 'contagion type interactional response'", this last item an expression of the diseased organism devalued role.

Within hospital settings, devalued classes are already gravely at risk (Wolfensberger, 1992b). In any institution of care people who are dying are at risk, especially if they embody another devalued characteristic as well as dying. Corley and Goren's (1998, pp 106-9) analysis of the types of patients stigmatised by nurses and the responses of nurses to such patients refers to a wide range of studies, including Kelly and May (1982), DeVellis et al (1984), Baer and Lowery (1987), Olbrisch and Levenson (1991), Carveth (1995) and Duffy (1995). Citing Baer and Lowery (1987), Corley and Goren (1998, p 107) indicate that the preferred (that is, valued) patient of student nurses is one who is "male, tidy, ambulatory, cheerful and communicative, and who ... [shows] some appreciation for their help". Patients whom student nurses judge as not to blame for their own pain are also preferred (Corley and Goren, 1998, pp 106-9). Nurses will tend to devalue patients exhibiting the opposite characteristics. Evidence confirms this. Grouping together the patient types stigmatised by nurses in the various studies and contexts discussed by Corley and Goren (1998, pp 106-9), nurses, broadly speaking, tend to stigmatise lesbians, patients with AIDS, people with psychiatric conditions, homeless people, suicidal people, women who choose abortion, people with alcohol abuse issues, sexual abuse perpetrators, patients with a disability and those patients who fail to comply or those who are simply not liked by the nurse. These findings concerning the 'dark side of nursing' (Jameton, 1992) sound a serious warning when nursing is supposedly the human, caring side of hospital care that compensates for the impersonal medical side. These findings reinforce the reality and gravity of the risks faced presently by devalued classes from hospital care, and by inference from palliative care through its nursing/medical dominance and institutional management. If the 'dark side of nursing' has transferred into palliative care nursing, which eventuality seems unavoidable, then the reality of palliative care may be very different from its image. For devalued classes especially, care in general and palliative care specifically may be as harmful as Corley and Goren's (1998) discussion suggest. Concerning hospital care for people with a disability, Corley and Goren (1998, p 109) note that "Deegan (1990) called the damage done to disabled patients by dehumanising and depersonalising care spirit breaking".

The factors presented by Corley and Goren (1998, pp 105-6) to explain the 'dark side of nursing' also reinforce the gravity of the problem. These factors are categorised into three groups:

- the ethical explanations – "nurses' lack of ethical consciousness of their use of coercive intervention", a lack of advocacy education and skills, and the "lack of a caring ethic" (Corley and Goren, 1998, pp 105-6, citing Tronto, 1993);
- the psychological explanation – lack of relationship with the patient;
- the organisational explanation that "group norms and processes may constrain the nurse's behaviour" (Corley and Goren, 1998, pp 105-6, citing Johnson and Webb, 1995).

Many authors from early on, for example Sudnow (1967) in respect of terminal and emergency care, have demonstrated the positive correlation between social value and quality of care and there seems little reason to suspect that human services, especially institutions, have changed.

The following more detailed explanation of the stereotypical devalued roles of SRV, from Chapter Four, shows how devalued stereotypes work together in relation to people who are dying specifically. People who are dying are seen as:

- *The holy innocent* – the idealised, romanticised roles as special or very special people; heroic, heroic virtue, close to God; especially blessed or wise; incapable of deceit, wrongdoing or self-interest; connected to *the once-again child* – since many people who are dying are also old, the infantilisation of older people in its many forms is naturally commonly applied.
- *The sick person, diseased organism/contagion* – the "'sick' 'patient' who, after 'diagnosis', is given 'treatment' or 'therapy' for his 'disease' in a 'clinic' or 'hospital' by 'doctors' who carry primary administrative and human management responsibility, assisted by a hierarchy of 'paramedical' personnel and 'therapists', all this hopefully leading to a 'cure'"(Wolfensberger, 1972, p 22).

- *The object of pity* – as in the sick person role the "pitied person is likely to be held blameless for his condition and perhaps unaccountable for his behaviour" (Wolfensberger, 1972, p 20); the 'deserving' person, the 'good cause'; connected to *the burden of charity role* where others feel a duty to care and may resent the obligation (Wolfensberger, 1998, p 15).
- *The dying/already dead/as good as dead* – placing people prematurely into the dying role, or seen as "having 'outlived their usefulness', may be related to as if they had already died, or had never existed" (Wolfensberger, 1998, p 16).

The *other/alien* role is also commonly connected to the *menace* role (for example, that he/she is no longer him/herself or scary) and to the *sub-human/non-human* role (for example, that he/she is just a vegetable now, better off dead).

Shifting these devalued role expectancies that become self-fulfilling prophecies requires the coherent promotion of valued images. For example, the burden of charity and object of pity roles are encouraged by intermingling philanthropy and volunteer support with care, and by using pitiful images of people who are dying in fund-raising campaigns. The holy innocent role is encouraged by religious connotations in care such as using religious motifs or inspirational words in service literature. Images of 'blameless' people who are dying looking gratefully at kind carers convey the once-again child role and holy innocent role. The already dead role and image is encouraged by institutionalising people who are dying with people who are very soon to be dead, or by funeral companies sponsoring palliative care services. Sponsorship of palliative care education by pharmaceutical companies conveys the sick person role. Situating a palliative care service in/near a nursing home would tend to ascribe the already dead role to both nursing home and palliative care users. Institutionalisation conveys the 'other' role and the menace role, needing to be isolated or secluded.

As another pervasive example of interrelated role stereotyping, the addition of the term 'therapy' to many forms of activity, such as massage, music, art and recreation as well as complementary therapies and grief therapy, conveys the sick person role. In palliative day care, one index lists 60-70 mostly everyday activities, excluding the various kinds of complementary therapy, under the heading 'creative therapies' (Bray, 1996, pp 198-221). And, as Wolfensberger (1975, p 14) puts it, the focus on "music, arts, crafts, parties, picnics and worship (eg chapel on the grounds)" conveys the object of pity model which "strives to bestow 'happiness'" via non-verbal, communal or creative forms of stimulation or expression.

Sensory therapy or stimulation rooms are a weird example, borrowed from the *snoezelen* (Dutch: *snuffeln*, sniff; *doezelen*, doze) (International Snoezelen Association, 2006: www.isna.de/index2e.html) of the intellectual disability services sector. The 'sensory suite' at the Prince and Princess of Wales Hospice's Day Care Centre (Prince and Princess of Wales Hospice, 2006) is an example. People who are dying should be supported to access the normal forms of sensory stimulation that most of us enjoy. The service system could be charged with trying to mask the dreadful impoverishment of experience produced by devaluation and institutional care with decorative, mystifying and spectacular diversions. The grand gesture is prominent in the paradigm of care, being used to delude devalued classes that society does care and to win status and respectability for benefactors/providers through demonstrating their charity. The institutional model can do nothing about the impoverishment of experience and the social isolation caused by institutional approaches. These are necessary accompaniments to its modus operandi. All an institutional model can do is substitute for the ordinary, real life of which it has deprived a person, replacing that life and its richness with weird imitations of reality and a relentless invention of faddish new ways to impoverish experience.

Simulating the real world devalues people, often through an overprotective intention, by denying them the real risks, challenges and opportunities of living that a valued person uses to enrich life and to grow. The hospice chapel or the palliative care service's library or the hospice garden or the palliative care service's relaxation, social or bereavement groups are all examples of the institutional model's simulation of the real world. Indeed the religio-therapeutic, hospice community – a 'counterfeit' community to use McKnight's (1995) term – itself substitutes for the community of origin but denies both the risks and opportunities that can occur only within that real community. The community of origin cannot learn how to live normally or naturally with people who are dying by visiting a hospice because the artificial, segregated community constructs everything abnormally and artificially, by definition. Hospice visitors can only imitate the abnormal impositions on ways of interrelating that have to obtain within a paid artificial community, whose uniformity in hospice cultural prescriptions is almost total, especially relative to the diversity of the community of origin.

Pet therapy is a useful, but relatively trivial, example to illustrate the way the institutional model of care can distort even the most common sense of propositions into a therapeutic mockery of the real thing. It is common sense to understand that people can respond to animals, and vice versa, and that this exchange can be rewarding. In the hospice, the valued social role of pet owner is denied and replaced with a simulation of the real role. The person receiving care is provided with the hospice's pet to enjoy without the responsibilities and risks of pet ownership, without the shared, deep commitment only attainable from the relationship between pet and guardian. If people own their own pets, then it would be more role-valorising for either the hospice to allow residents to bring their own pets with them, just as people can bring other possessions, or to design a service model that allows people to remain at home with their pet. The service system can pretend benevolence by developing strange service adaptations or substitutes that try to compensate for the losses it imposes. The staff and institution are then thought to be responsive to individual needs and to possess a special understanding of such needs, a special understanding that alone can appreciate the benefit of such strange service adaptations that mock the lost life.

Weird adaptations to replace the loss of people's own pets become increasingly ridiculous the more the institutional model is stretched beyond its institutional setting. The Pets As Therapy (PAT) charity, founded in 1983 in the UK (PAT, 2003) brings pets, which are not the residents' pets, to visit hospital, hospice or nursing home aiming to provide therapy through bringing happiness and comfort, according to PAT (PAT, 2003). The institutional model thus keeps up its claim to meeting every possible need and so to being the best, ultimate and only solution.

Unconsciousness of the processes of devaluation allows pet therapy to be claimed an achievement in humanising care. As Race (1999, p 51) notes, pet therapy conveys animalistic messages about devalued people, that is, it conveys the sub-human organism role. The use of pets in a hospice to make people who are dying happy or to comfort them also conveys the object of pity role. That it is called pet *therapy* (or pet/animal assisted *therapy*) conveys the devalued sick person role. The inescapable deindividualisation intrinsic to institutional approaches is again evident because some people hate animals and have very negative responses to them, even being terrified of them or just being allergic to them. The use of hospice animals, a part of hospice culture, demands a deindividualisation of care. If a valued person in his/her private home were to be convinced of the value of 'pet therapy', then the person would simply buy a pet or buy in resources sufficient enough to keep him/herself and his/her pet well cared for at home.

Despite all the contortions of the institutional model to try to meet individual needs and to try to compensate for the loss of roles and community that institutionalisation demands, the real solution can be found in a spot that proves several key points about institutional models. These important points are: institutional models deny alternatives; institutional models promote solutions that are completely inappropriate for socially devalued people; and without institutions new more appropriate alternatives can develop. An alternative solution is the Pets Are Wonderful Support (PAWS) organisation that seeks to keep animals with their guardians for as long as possible by, for example, offering financial support, providing care and grooming for animals, driving people to veterinarians or groomers, and fostering the animals in their own homes during their guardian's hospital admission (PAWS, 2003). This service adaptation is relatively appropriate since it promotes the maintenance of the valued role of pet owner/guardian.

Besides the alternative that such a model represents to the devaluing institutional conceptions of pet therapy or the hospice pet, the critical fact is that these agencies originated as HIV/AIDS-specific support services. People with HIV/AIDS generally do not use generic hospice care for a variety of reasons, so this group of people must create an alternative solution outside the institutional model. Because social devaluation is such a risk for people with HIV/AIDS, it is not surprising that this solution is relatively role valorising and so protective against such devaluation. PAWS indicates strikingly that increasing home support options and adopting a 'whatever-it-takes' approach to maintaining the valued role (at home) should be the alternative that is developed, rather than wasting resources on strange adaptations of the pity-charitable model such as PAT. The PAWS example shows that the institutional way is not 'the only way'. If an institution is not built, or is not accessible for some reason, the community, if guided by stigmatised groups within it, invents highly individualised, more role-valorising alternatives.

Competency and image enhancement (Wolfensberger, 1998, pp 62-82)

The ideology of institutional settings and models holds that the acquisition of pseudo-competencies can replace, supersede or be of more value than competencies developed within the normal community. Under this ideology, the acquisition of new 'therapeutic' competencies, such as openness, intimacy and emotional expressiveness, or 'spiritual' competencies, such as hope, security, peace or acceptance, justifies or compensates for the loss of existing competencies that institutionalisation demands. Saunders (1977, 1995) describes such competency achievements as typical, although not occurring in every case, and also sometimes as occurring "with surprising speed" (Saunders, 1995, p xiv). By institutionalisation, growth or other experiences are denied their chance for expression within the normal patterns of living of the person who is dying. While this disregard for the sense of place and context of the individual is significant, the essential problem concerning these new competencies is that they are predicated on the loss of any number of pre-existing, often context-specific competencies along with the valued roles these genuine competencies enable. An attendant problem is that it cannot readily be determined to what extent such new 'competencies' are a reflection of the artificial intensification of experience in a hospice and the events witnessed therein, which occurs on top of an impoverishment of one's ordinary living experiences upon institutionalisation and the numerous losses involved in losing one's home.

If the acquisition of new competencies is predicated on the loss of others, then it is very difficult to know to what extent this acquisition is an expression or consequence of that loss. To what extent is a new competency a clutching at the only straw left in the face of tragedy upon tragedy; or a mere filling of the void to reassert some identity or purpose; or a believing and cherishing since almost all of what was believed or held dear has been lost; or a reinvention of self according to what is being culturally prescribed; or an untransferrable effect only able to be manifested within the therapeutic community? Even miraculous transformations cannot justify imposing, through institutionalisation, losses on people who are soon to lose their entire corporeal life. These are vital issues for palliative care that sees so much good in modelling by the therapeutic community and so much therapeutic and spiritual value in group dying in a segregated community.

Since palliative care's inception only one very small, inconclusive and problematic study, Honeybun et al (1992), has made an even rudimentary attempt to examine whether group dying is experienced as a good thing by hospice inpatients. There is a considerable body of anecdote and rhetoric endorsing group dying. However, Clark and Seymour (1999, pp 54–5) refer to apparently worrying evidence from Seale and Addington-Hall's (1994, 1995) very large study across 20 health districts in England. Clark and Seymour (1999, p 55) report the astonishing conclusion of the study: "spending time in a hospice in the last year of life increases the likelihood of a request for euthanasia"

– 8.8% of people who spent some time in a hospice compared to 3.6% of people who spent no time in a hospice. Respondents for people who had some care in a hospice were 1.7 times more likely than respondents for people spending no time in a hospice to feel it would have been better if the person who was dying had died earlier. Although Clark and Seymour (1999, p 55) specify some possible confounding factors in the data and some later speculation by Seale et al (1997) that hypothesises hospice's open awareness to dying as a relevant factor, these results appear to raise disturbing questions about the effects of being in a hospice, as well as the effects of hospice culture and its open awareness context. SRV theory argues that devaluation has an enormous range of negative effects on people by internalising this devaluation and by being oppressed by it.

The loss of competencies escalates upon institutionalisation because of the impoverishment and artificiality of institutional life, and because new residents imitate existing residents, who will usually possess a lower level of competency. An inexorable decline to the lowest common denominator of behaviour and competency follows. Acceleration to the highest levels of compliance, dependency, and standardisation of competency and behaviour also follows. In the hospice or hospital, people imitate other residents who have already conformed to the hospice or hospital culture. As a result, people are, for example, likely to not understand privacy as they would at home, or dignity, or the right to have intimate conversations in absolute privacy and confidentiality. The enormous power of any institutional culture to prescribe behaviour is a barrier to genuine change from imitation of practitioner's modelling since its authority tends to overwhelm critical attitudes and conform individual differences.

Having explored competency enhancement a little, the discussion now examines the enhancement of social imagery. Race (1999, pp 110-18) explores general examples concerning social imagery. Derived from the PASSING manual (Program Analysis of Service Systems' Implementation of Normalisation Goals) of Wolfensberger and Thomas (1983), Race's (1999, pp 115-18) table lists the key media, such as service name and setting, by which images are conveyed in human services.

The names of hospice and palliative care services can be classified into four groups: the religious, the sentimentally idealised, the descriptive and the personalised. Personalised organisational names, which could include a benefactor's name such as the Prince and Princess of Wales Hospice, or the name of a significant service user, convey images of charity and the goodness of the cause. Personalised names also convey any associations particular to the name, such as the cultural specificity denoted by an Anglo–Saxon name or child–like images denoted by a child's name.

Religious mystification, cultures, ideologies and images are conveyed by religious names such as 'Hospice of Genesis', 'Amitabha Hospice Service' or the many saint–named hospices. Sentimentally idealised names convey sentimental and idealised images of death and dying, often implying the resolution of the problem of death and dying, as do the religious names. Moreover, a unique kind of goodness or nobility is conveyed. In the words of numerous hospices, hospice provides "a special kind of caring" (for example, Southeast Hospice, 2006) or even "a very special kind of caring" (for example, Covenant Hospice, 2007) or "very special care" (St Christopher's Hospice, 2003b). Examples of sentimentally idealised names include 'Hospice Hands', 'Life Doors Hospice' and 'Alive Hospice'. All these titles imply a mystification of hospice care and death and dying as something beyond the ordinary, as do the religious names. As Lofland (1978) points out, paradoxical titles like 'Alive Hospice' particularly convey the idea of mystification and the resolution of the problem of death by implying that hospice possesses a wisdom beyond the conventional.

Often hospice logos or the quasi–religious paintings on walls, for example at St Christopher's Hospice (Saunders, 1977, p 175), convey the same message. Seale (1998, p 119) cites Froggatt and Walter's (1995) examination of hospice logos in remarking that "resolution of liminality is suggested" by these illustrations. Motifs such as doorway, window, flower and tree also convey the romantic idealisation of death (Seale, 1998), as do other common logos with suns, sunsets, birds, pathways, horizons, butterflies, hands, hearts or rural scenes.

The merely descriptive names convey a relatively neutral image common to many valued services such as medical clinics, simply describing the location and nature of the service. Necessary access information is provided, such as the type/location of service, without any kind of mystification, idealisation, sentimentality or personification, at least via the services' titles. 'Connecticut Hospice' is an example. Although usually an image that is relatively image neutral will be the most valuing as a title, the culturally valued analogue specific to the area and culture should be used as a guide.

Devaluing images can derive from the building itself and the history of the building. The medical history of many hospice inpatient facilities associates the sick person role with people who are dying and constructs palliative care as essentially a medical/nursing endeavour. Carey (1986) examines 21 US inpatient hospice facilities from an architectural viewpoint. (Less than 20% have descriptive names.) Eleven hospices were formerly used for medical-related purposes. (One of these was formerly a mental rehabilitation unit, thereby associating people who are dying with those with a psychiatric disability, and devaluing both groups.) Two hospices were formerly elementary schools conveying the role of child. Four other hospices were sited in or adjoining hospitals. One was located in a university campus and another in a living centre, seemingly a day care centre. The juxtaposition of people who are dying with people with a disability via day care centres increases the devaluation of both groups. The remaining three facilities were freestanding, new (or always had been) hospices and one of these was classified as a 'pre-hospice skilled nursing facility'. Only one of the 21 facilities, the one in the university, was situated in a building whose history attached valuing images to people who are dying, unless that building happened to be the old zoology or psychology building, for example.

Philanthropic images abound in palliative care and reinforce the extra-special worthiness of the cause and the staff, and reinforce the rest of the burden of charity role. The Prince and Princess of Wales Hospice in Glasgow is a prime example. The online literature of this hospice states the perennial "it is our belief that death is a natural part of living" (Prince and Princess of Wales Hospice, 2003) yet almost every image connected with the hospice is exceptional. These include its name, the scale of its building and its purpose-built day care centre, its many shops spread around Glasgow and its dramatic connection with Princess Diana and her 'unnatural' death. The key image association in this example is the respectability and nobility of palliative care, and also its regal authority. The privileged class's duty to provide care and the devalued class's gratitude for this gift is also pre-eminently imaged.

The shops associated with the hospice might be expected to be at the top end of the market. However, the extremely grand and noble image associations from Princess Diana contrast starkly with the image associations of the shops, which all sell second-hand clothing, books and bric-a-brac, and unwanted furniture (Prince and Princess of Wales Hospice, 2003). Raising funds from discarded items is a typical way in which devalued people are cast into the role of useless waste, as Race (1999, p 56) notes. Although some highly valued institutions, such as English private schools, might also use charity shops, the extremely high social status of these schools/students readily absorbs the impact of any devaluing effects from associations of the 'waste/rubbish' or 'burden of charity' devalued role. However, for people at risk of social devaluation such associations would have a disproportionately negative effect on overall status. Wolfensberger (1998) demonstrates that highly valued status absorbs devaluing tendencies and can even transform a devalued characteristic into a highly prized one in exceptional circumstances. In the case of this hospice, valueless waste and poverty/ charity image associations are juxtaposed dramatically with those of the greatest wealth, value and privilege. This juxtaposition of imagery further intensifies the rightness of the 'gift relation' (Porter, 1989) between the privileged and the devalued. The clash of image juxtapositions serves to intensify the message that the connection between the hospice and its royal patrons is unnatural or extraordinary. With a patron whose 'unnatural' death created such an emotional outpouring, and with so great a conflict in imagery, the mystique of palliative care as something extra special and noble is amplified.

Conflicting images convey confusion, at the very least. Conflicting, confusing image associations, together with the implied deference and awe surrounding palliative care, convey that the subject is just too profound or special to understand, beyond the grasp of the normal person. Only the most 'special' people, such as Princess Diana and those who work in palliative care, could grasp death and dying and react normally or appropriately.

The other side of the coin, the benefactor's self-interest, is ignored. Princess Diana accepted the gift of the hospice as a young woman relatively new to royal life. The image associations of palliative care add to her a maturity, authority and compassion beyond her years and experience. This is not to question in any way the personal motives of Princess Diana, but to indicate that the institutional model of care serves the interests of benefactors, including their political and social interests. Non-institutional services cannot serve these interests. A royal patron offering his/her sympathy to a ward full of people who are dying and their grateful families, as well as his/her appreciation to the 'very special' staff, creates an indelible and magical media image. The same patron visiting the private home of one person who is dying would convey an altogether less compelling and noteworthy picture. In the same way, donating funds to a visiting palliative care nursing service to employ staff is very different, from a public relations' viewpoint, to donating funds to build a new palliative day care centre or a new ward for a hospice.

The financing of palliative care services, including fund-raising, is a key area in which social imagery plays an important role in constructing the messages a palliative care service conveys. Race (1999, p 59) indicates that "appeal activities that rely on the presentation of suffering people or actually use devalued people themselves again reinforce the pity role, as do various setting features that emphasise the motivation of the staff is out of pity, especially those with religious overtones". Since the religious overtones and the religious motivation of staff are so strong in palliative care, the object of pity role is strongly promoted. Financing from general revenue implies the rectitude of society's obligation to care for people who are dying and, in so doing, denies the pity role propagated by fundraising. The 'begging letter', which seeks donations to charitable organisations, is known as such for good reason.

Palliative care abounds with many totally inappropriate image juxtapositions, including in fund-raising. For example, a brick can be purchased, that is the devalued (dying) person as insensate object, to go into the hospice memorial footpath and can be inscribed with the name of the deceased (Haven Hospice, 2006). The culturally valued analogues for memorialisation are the cemetery, private home and individual monument, the monument to group dying in war being the key exception. Even if it could be justified somehow that it was appropriate to memorialise at a hospice service, memorialisation is corrupted by using it to raise funds. This could only ever be considered appropriate for a devalued class of people. Few would seek to use the memorialisation of a war hero or president as a way to raise funds. Such fund-raising memorialisation also devalues isolated or poor people who die at the hospice, because they may have no one to buy them a brick or may have families who cannot afford a brick.

Sponsorship is another area where negative image juxtapositions abound, for example, a fast food chain sponsoring cancer services for children and drug companies sponsoring medical education seminars in palliative care. In these examples, the direct payoffs include increased income, for sponsor and service, and status, compassion and credibility for sponsors by associating themselves with the fight against cancer and the conquest of the unpalatable aspects of dying. Palliative care services use fund-raising to inculcate hospice culture. This can occur, for example, by the sale of butterfly badges (religious connotations) or second-hand goods (charitable connotations) or seeking donations from bequests and the connections of the deceased (gratitude expectation).

A lack of recognition of the dynamics and relevance of social imagery riddles the literature of palliative care, for example Fisher (1991, p 8), or almost any of the online literature. This ignorance of the processes of devaluation allows for gross misinterpretations of the SRV theme to compensate for devalued status via positive images. Hospices should not be overly serious, drab or morose environments, since these are the stereotypical negative images surrounding death and dying. Neither should they be the hilarious, circus-type environments encouraged by the work of people like 'Patch Adams' ('Patch Adams', 1998). The nature of institutional models demands service adaptations are distorted into bizarre parodies of normal life. It is only the institutional nature of the model of care that drives serious people like Adams to such lengths, to try to balance the size and intensity of the tragedy of group dying or group hospitalisation with some kind of humanity. The hospice itself was driven to the lengths of creating its own institution to replace the dehumanising approach of hospitalised dying with a more humane ethic.

The abnormality of the institutional model necessitates abnormal adaptations of the service system, as has been said. If a role-valorising approach is adopted, then the system adapts normatively. There is no need for a 'Patch Adams' when people are dying at home. People can go to a comedy show, or to the circus, or hire a clown whenever they want, or watch hilarious movies day after day. In the hospital, or hospice/ palliative care ward, or psychiatric ward, or nursing home, or day care centre, or homeless shelter, or drug detoxification facility a 'Patch Adams' becomes a necessity. However, under the institutional model applied in non-acute contexts, a 'Patch Adams' would not be 'special' enough. His approach would have to be adapted to become extremely institutional, to become something deeply devaluing and bizarre, so that the institution, perversely, could claim its title as ultimate repository of care and expertise. The most devaluing option is the development of the 'very special' expertise of the institution's own in-house laughter therapy team. Sadly, hospice laughter therapy teams already exist (for example, Hospice of the Florida Suncoast, 2006) and the true message of 'Patch Adams'' compassion is thereby mocked and misunderstood.

From an SRV-based perspective, the institutional model is inherently devaluing since it exhibits intractable paradoxes in its way of caring. The paradoxes of models of care with significant institutional expression are more evident or easily grasped when understood in relation to institutions themselves. Nevertheless, SRV theory emphasises that devaluation can occur anywhere. The paradoxes that follow should be understood mostly in the broader context of institutional approaches to care, equally relevant to community care as to care in an institution. For example, while people who are dying are grouped together in hospices, people can also be grouped together at community-based palliative care services for such things as meditation groups or social occasions. And specialist palliative care teams, whether in hospices or in private homes, tend to provide the vast majority of direct care themselves, a characteristic feature of the institutional approach.

SRV proponents have identified a mindset of false beliefs and claims that have supported the continuation of institutional care for people with an intellectual disability in the face of criticism from normalisation from the 1960s, and later from SRV. The term 'benevolent institution myth' (Harris, 1995) encapsulates this mindset. In summary, this mindset believes that institutions of care are both benevolent and necessary, providing ultimate, total care for devalued people. The existence of institutions 'proves' their necessity and 'proves' that the needs being serviced are so drastic as to be only serviceable via institutional care. Institutions are, therefore, self-validating. The never-ending litany of exposés about institutional negligence and abuse, from every type of institution without exception, disproves claims of the benevolence of institutional approaches. Nevertheless, the 'benevolent institution myth' remains very powerful and superficially convincing.

Some key elements of the 'anti-institutionalisation' argument are brought together with respect to intellectual disability services in Ferleger and Boyd (1980) and Laski (1980) in their discussions of a lawsuit against a Pennsylvanian institution in 1977. The court "declared the existence of the institution was unconstitutional", concluding that the institution "was not providing, and could never provide, that minimally adequate habilitation that occurs only in a normalized setting" (Ferleger and Boyd, 1980, p 153). Wolfensberger (1976a, 1976b) also contains further background concerning the anti-institutionalisation idea. Wolfensberger (1976b) can find no "programmatic, ideological or fiscal grounds [that can] salvage" the institutional model. In the process Wolfensberger (1976b) challenges the 'economies of scale' (Porter, 1989, p 163) argument in relation to intellectual disability institutions in the US. Wolfensberger (1976b, p 425) states: "the dogma that we cannot afford to scrap our institutional system because of financial reasons is almost universally accepted. I submit this dogma is a myth", and he goes on to cite supporting evidence from the Presidential Committee on Mental Retardation.

The case that institutions are not benevolent involves one qualification. Historically, some institutions have been relatively benevolent, at least for a time. Since hospices reduce the abuses of hospitalised dying, hospices are relatively benevolent toward people who are dying compared to hospitals. A number of other reform movements have done the same, replicated the institutional model and established separate, specialised institutions so as to insulate the reform from corrupting influences and develop the modality of care.

This is entirely understandable. The institutional model should be regarded, however, as a rudimentary or initial formalisation of social organisation, evolution beyond this form being necessary to moderate the social devaluation inherent in institutional management. This evolution is the subject of Chapter Six.

Paradoxes of institutional models of care

Exclude and include paradox

This paradox indicates that institutional approaches exclude while aiming to include. Segregation of people at risk of social devaluation stigmatises and distinguishes the inmate from those outside, the typical valued citizen. Grouping people who are dying together has a multiplier effect, compounding their social devaluation and exclusion. One person who is dying in his/her own home is unremarkable. A whole group of people who are dying is a compelling and tragic scene. Some might contend that it is an inspiring and 'very special' scene. The social analogues of group dying are, for example, war, natural disaster, the extermination of devalued groups, plague and famine. These analogues disprove the romantic imagery believed to be conveyed by group dying.

A corollary to this paradox concerns the level of accountability institutional models of care are able to achieve when people have been excluded from their normal community and their social roles. Institutional models reduce accountability while aiming to increase accountability. Institutions through their respectability, status and authority, claim a high level of accountability. Social approval often attaching to caring staff also promotes the same belief, and the belief that such staff members do no harm. Obligatory gratitude demanded for the provision of institutional care makes complaining seem improper. The size and authority of the institution make complaining difficult and also tend to make it easier to hide harmful activities by individuals. An institution commonly closes ranks to defend itself from claims of negligence or poor service. Complex bureaucratic processes in large institutions also make complaining difficult. Problem staff might be changed but the institutional culture remains the same. Changes made to address wrongs decline in effectiveness over time, and reform is often merely in name.

Institutions are commonly like mazes or rabbit warrens. Institutions are always disorienting and it is usually hard to find where to go. Institutions construct a series of physical boundaries that have to be crossed before reaching those sections where people receive care. The institution shuts away from public scrutiny what actually goes on. Some of the ever-present influences of institutions on residents and visitors alike are: isolation, disempowerment, fear, alienation, disorientation, confusion, awe and dread. The threatening aura of any institution of care, and the threat embodied in the dire conditions being handled within it, cautions against approaching, and cautions against questioning what goes on inside because dire circumstances imply that dire measures should be taken. Inmates and visitors alike are so overwhelmed by the institution that they do not expect to understand what is taking place there.

Inside the institution visitors, as well as inmates, must obey the institutional requirements and protocols, often without understanding the rationale for such restrictions or directions. Institutional mystique and visitors' lack of understanding about what is taking place and why, increase the hesitance of visitors to make judgements about what they see or are told. The institution becomes a provider of secret business. Sanitised care in sanitised environments by standardised means secretes or masks the disturbing aspects of care and disturbing behaviours, as a number of authors have noted, for example Charmaz (1980). Because many of one's rights are given up upon institutionalisation, visitors can assume a 'you just have to get used to it' attitude, and so themselves urge residents to comply and not complain. Whatever the institution does becomes beyond question. Compliance in institutional care is almost absolute. Since residents lose the power and rights they held in their own home, and since the power of the institution is so astronomical in comparison, institutional power will be abused and will be abused significantly, as the almost daily reports of institutional abuses testify. Since the institution can and usually does control everything about the person's life, the potential for abuse far exceeds anything that could occur in a person's own home, especially since no other services act as safeguards.

Increase and decrease fear paradox

This paradox indicates that institutional approaches increase fear while aiming to decrease fear. The exclusion of the outside world from institutions of care and the ultimate or total treatment conducted within them create both the institution and the devalued condition of inmates as threatening and abnormal. The community is excluded by everything about the institution, including the messages it sends about its inmates and what goes on within its walls. Exclusion exacerbates the fear of difference. Although aiming to reduce the fear of inmates and the community, by claiming to be able to handle any situation relating to the 'dire' condition, the institution actually increases the fear surrounding both the person and the condition, not to mention the institution itself.

Grouping devalued people together affirms the myth of the abnormality of difference and the fear associated with it. Service users, family and friends dread entering the institution because of what it signifies and because of what happens there. The community avert their eyes in dread and pity when they walk past. Walking past a private home where a person is dying evokes an entirely different response. The mere existence of an institution for devalued people implants and exaggerates stigmatisation, fear, awe and the mystique of taboo in the minds of service users and the community.

Institutions create a devalued social characterisation or stereotype of those using the service. More precisely, this characterisation is a caricature because it is a falsification that exaggerates what is most different or devalued about the inmates, which is their dying in the case of palliative care. Inmates lose all individuality to passers-by, becoming merely a mass of identical dying faces, in identical beds, in numerous standardised rooms or wards, off identical corridors served by numerous standardised staff. People who are dying become an homogeneous class of pitiable people. Dying in a private home, individuality and the meaning of the loss of individuality become intensely imaged in the minds of passers-by, the community and residents themselves. A whole range of alternative meanings is expressed concerning suffering, sacrifice, love and loss, for example. In an institution all these meanings are distorted, if only because their manifestation occurs in a context that is an abnormal expression of the typical, valued living patterns of a person and the community.

An institution such as a hospice also confirms just how grave the problem is. Every person with the devalued condition becomes a potential candidate to have the most extreme expression of the condition, no matter the likelihood of this occurring, since the institution engenders the belief that the condition itself is so extreme that only institutional care is able to cope with it. The common expectation becomes that every person with the devalued condition does or will require institutional care, since the condition already is or will become dire, irrespective of the actual proportion of people likely to exhibit the most severe forms of the condition. Since the devalued condition known as dying always ends in death, it is 'certain' that the condition will become 'dire', although many people die quite peacefully without any dire clinical circumstances eventuating. As a result the community's tolerance of difficulties arising from the condition reduces and, over time, institutionalisation occurs for people with milder and milder instances of the condition. The increased fear of the condition, caused by dealing with it through institutional care, means people also tend to be institutionalised at increasingly earlier stages, and that, over time, a greater proportion will be institutionalised. The community becomes less tolerant of and responsive to the difference known as dying.

All and no options paradox

This paradox indicates that institutional approaches reduce options by aiming to provide all options. Centralising expertise and facilities in institutions reduces access to those distant from them. Demographic profiles change, the locations of institutions cannot. An all-embracing specialist facility implies that only a reduced, inferior standard of care is available in alternative settings. The choice becomes all or nothing – complete security from choosing the total care of the institution or terrible danger from choosing the inferior care of alternative settings. To what extent are people who are dying reluctant or scared to die at home because they feel they might need the level of care the *existence* of hospices implies only a hospice can provide? To what extent are families reluctant or scared to care for people who are dying at home because families feel they could never provide the level of care the *existence* of hospices implies only a hospice can provide?

Again, accountability is reduced by providing all or most care options from the one source. A lack of competition for market share encourages complacency. Accountability can readily be compromised if there is no economic incentive to be accountable. If there are no alternatives, to what can the standard of institutional care be compared? The ordinary citizen or inmate cannot make any comparison of quality of care because he/she does not have the necessary knowledge and experience to judge institutional processes. With a variety of service options and organisations serving the same clientele, the web of options increases the scrutiny of care and service users' ability to choose appropriate support options.

Solving/not solving all the problems paradox

This paradox indicates that the aim of institutions is to solve all the problems regarding a certain condition, yet institutions are never big enough or expert enough to solve all the problems. Institutional approaches keep spreading and increasing in specialisation, and keep promising indefinite progress until the final elimination of the problems of dying, for example, yet problems remain no matter how big or expert the institutions and specialists become. Palliative care teams increase in the number of specialist workers without any clear rationale about how to determine what is appropriate in an ideal sense (for example, Hockley and Mowatt, 1996). The perennial specialist versus generalist debate, noted by Robbins (1998), and the ever-increasing scope of palliative care nursing practice illustrate this paradox of the institutional model. Seeking to be the ultimate repository of expertise, this model finds no way to rationalise this need to be 'everything to everybody', with the amount of care required (for example, Fisher, 1996, p 248). Only cost containment or mere availability act as a basis for determining whether specialist or generalist staff should provide care. Concerning the scope of nursing practice, both its breadth and depth continue to increase, apparently without questioning the appropriateness or significance of nurses providing such all-encompassing care. Yates (1998, pp 109-11) and Parsons (1998, pp 265-6) are just two of the authors who raise some of the problems concerning, respectively, the breadth and depth requirements of nursing expertise.

Even the arguments concerning how to determine the appropriate use of volunteers have no theoretical or ethical basis, and tend to reduce to appeals to availability and expedience. Relf and Couldrick (1988) use the deprofessionalisation argument in advocating that volunteers should deliver bereavement care because grief is not an illness. According to this principle, all pre-death grief should also be handled by volunteers. Since nurses dominate palliative care, pre-death grief will be handled, for the most part, by nurses, which conveys the image that pre-death grief is an illness. "Bereavement support is provided in the main by volunteers ... the Macmillan Nurses [specialist cancer and palliative care nurses] may give support to a small number of families" (Relf and Couldrick, 1988, p 133). The criterion of normalising grief, therefore, is easily sidelined by the overriding, medical model assumption that specialist (nursing) expertise is not needed for the standard majority of bereaved people and should be reserved for the more complex or needy 'small number of families'. This assumption is also a way to ration a limited availability of specialists. In other words, the limited availability of specialist nurses means this resource must be rationed, therefore volunteers should provide the vast bulk of bereavement support.

Saunders (1977) tries to make St Christopher's Hospice more home-like using deprofessionalisation in various forms and also instituting strange service adaptations that would seem highly unusual to the uninitiated, such as the school club on holidays or the playgroup all year round (Saunders, 1977, p 162). From an SRV-based perspective, adaptations like these are efforts to compensate for the losses caused by institutionalisation. These so-called 'community inclusion' approaches are a type of devaluation as well as deprofessionalisation, which is not just an expedient to ration resources or cut costs but is, more importantly, a means to cloak the artificialities of hospice life in the appearance of everyday ordinariness and normalcy. In this process of masking devaluation with unusual service adaptations, which are actually a counterfeit substitute for valued life, a new culture is formed incorporating these peculiar artificialities that become part of what then becomes known as hospice culture or its special way of caring. Saunders' compassion has to try to balance the devaluation of hospitalised approaches with some kind of adjustment to moderate their inhumanity. Unusual adaptations of hospital and institutional processes are developed to try to make the institution of the hospice more home-like, more community-like, more life-like and less devaluing. However, because the organisational form she chose is both religio-medical and institutional, these peculiar adaptations necessarily remain devaluing and perpetuate devaluation in relatively "harder-to-decipher forms", to use the term of Kristiansen et al (1999, p 450).

Randall and Downie (1999, p 25) go even further along the incoherent, deprofessionalisation path. Concerning all support for "anxiety, grief, loneliness, and general unhappiness", they call the belief that there are professional, psychosocial skills that can assist in these areas "a delusion". In this illustration and Relf and Couldrick's (1988), the marginalisation of psychosocial skills, knowledge and personnel within palliative care is very clear. Structuring volunteers into taking over most of the bereavement support allows nurses to colonise bereavement for the 'difficult cases' when these 'difficult cases' are one of the clearest examples of the roles that society expects psychosocial/spiritual specialists to perform.

The scope of nursing practice is a highly problematic issue in palliative care. Since nurses fulfil case management functions in palliative care the scope of nursing practice in palliative care expands into another complex field. Advocacy is a key aspect of the case management role. In respect of just the normal advocacy role of nurses, and not the more complex advocacy involved in case management, Corley and Goren (1998, p 105) note: "the nurse's advocacy role is relatively recent....Thus, nurses who have not been educated in advocacy may not have the skills to function as patient advocates". The inappropriateness of nurses acting as advocates is raised by Randall and Downie (1999), who recommend specifically excluding nurses from acting as advocates in palliative care because of the ethical impossibility of perhaps having to advocate against oneself when an advocate also provides direct care. Randall and Downie (1999) offer some grounds for determining appropriate palliative care practitioner duties in general, but only by further replicating the institutional, hospital/medical model. In this approach, generally the medical good of the person has primacy over every other benefit to the person. The institutional model of palliative care assumes that services' staff, who are predominantly nurses, should provide the vast majority of support. It is to be expected, therefore, that the expertise of specialist palliative care nursing can never be broad or deep enough.

Institutions can never be big enough. Spooner (1996, p 63) indicates that day care centres in Britain came about in palliative care because of increasing demands for hospice inpatient care and domiciliary services, as well as increasing costs. No ethical basis or rationale of appropriateness drives day care development. Day care centres are a replication of the institutional model, an institutional service adaptation forced to develop since hospices can never be big enough or wholly comprehensive. Hospices must then jettison services, in the case of day care predominantly respite care services, by sending out satellite mini-institutions. Day care centres are purely day hospices from an organisational viewpoint. Although day care has been the most rapidly growing area of palliative care in Britain in the 1990s, its effectiveness is unevaluated (Higginson, 1996, p 112). Higginson (1996) goes on to say that the need for evaluation is urgent since the only study in the literature, citing Macdonald and Macdonald (1992), rated day care the least useful of hospice options. It therefore seems clear that something other than usefulness in care or user/carer need is driving the explosion of the day care fad. Hospices aim to provide all care, to be everything to everyone, and so solve the problem of dying. When this becomes unfeasible, as it must, hospices can only jettison into mini-institutions some services, which will be those services, such as respite care or non-cancer services, which are least effective at promoting institutional agenda.

Institutional models are most quickly recognised by their range of services, which is usually very large, trying to provide for all needs from the one source, as demonstrated by the list of the 14 services that Spooner (1996, pp 63-4) believes palliative day centres can and should provide. Spooner's (1996) institutional kind of thinking believes it is appropriate for palliative day care to provide such services as hairdressing, complementary medicine or even medical care. A day care centre providing hairdressing and massage denies a person who is dying yet one more valued social role, that of local consumer, when a person could go to his/her own local hairdresser, or the hairdresser could come to the home of the person who is dying, or some other valuing alternative. Under the institutional day care model, local services, such as hairdressing, need make no adjustments that might be required, for example, to support access to its services for people who are dying. Local services have no opportunity to continue to value their valued consumer in the ways they have always done.

Doyle (1990, pp 5-6) is just one of those who discover dilemma upon dilemma when starting to explore how to service appropriately the needs of non-traditional hospice clients, such as those with AIDS or Alzheimer's disease. Clark and Seymour (1999, p 158) refer to UK policy initiatives that suggest that "similar services [to palliative care] should be developed for patients dying from diseases other than cancer", although the current evidence regarding any such integration shows "fragmentation" and a lack of fit in the "majority of cases". Should there be special AIDS hospices? Should the care of people with Alzheimer's disease be incorporated into an expanded intake for hospice care? A number of authors in Goldman (1998) raise the problems facing children who are dying in an institutional system that excludes their difference, which is simply that they are children who are dying rather than adults. Existing hospice institutions cannot individualise for children because these facilities collect adults together to die. And within specialised children's hospices/hospitals, the problem is that the particularity of each child's individual circumstances cannot be adequately met, such as the need for social contact with local friends.

Many other problems arise from the disruption caused by the rigid, distant location necessary for specialist institutions to be feasible economically. The system blames the person at risk of devaluation. People's needs are complex or too individual or too specialised to be met in any other way. The institutional model does not acknowledge its eradication of non-institutional alternatives nor its rigid organisational nature and, therefore, it will accept none of the responsibility. Under the institutional model, there can be no criteria, other than expedience, including availability of expertise, and cost to determine whether developments such as children's hospices, or illness-specialised hospices, or more generic hospices are appropriate. This must occur since the institutional model has no other way to address the need for individualisation other than specialisation through building more, bigger or different institutions, and through an ever-expanding scope of clinical practice.

Several authors in Goldman (1998) also raise the perennial problem about who are the appropriate personnel to service the great variety in needs. Towards a resolution of these difficulties, Baum (1998, p 11) suggests the importance of recognising a proper place for paediatric palliative care within the social organisation of palliative care, that is, to emphasise a subspecialty within the specialty of palliative care, with all the vast range of expertise relevant to this minority. Under this logic, since palliative care might also service people with psychiatric disorders or intellectual disabilities or HIV/AIDS or multiple sclerosis or cystic fibrosis or any number of other 'specialised' conditions and situations, specialisation upon specialisation can be the only answer, generating numerous subspecialties in either specialised hospices or some other institutional form. McEnhill (2004) raises this and other issues concerning palliative care provision to people with a disability.

Baum's (1998) type of thinking is based on the assumptions of the institutional medical model, which is unable to service all needs because it cannot individualise care. The gaps in, or more correctly, the exclusions by today's medical system, which is the most specialised and far-reaching system of care that there has ever been, demonstrate this point. Unless the organisation of the system is changed to centre on the home, there is no solution other than never-ending specialisation, and never-ending expansion of expertise and institution building. Relentless replication of the institutional model is the only option, until we look outside this model.

The institutional type of thinking of Doyle (1990) and Baum (1998), for example, appears to be asking: how are people with relatively complex needs, or needs outside the traditional range of hospice, best serviced? People with needs outside the traditional range are in danger of being victimised by the way these questions are framed, for example by these needs being called complex, different or specialised. Questions such as these assume that these needs must, can and should be met within the institutional model of palliative care that itself is responsible, via its construction, for the exclusion and devaluation of non-traditional needs in the first place.

Doyle (1990) is quite correct to recognise that something akin to hospice care can and should be used to service all chronic conditions rather than hospice simply serving people with cancer. Bradshaw (1996, p 412) too sees hospice care as able to be applied to all incurable conditions, indeed able to be applied to *"anyone* who needs care" (original emphasis). In suspecting that society will see hospices as an appropriate institution for the care of people with Alzheimer's disease, and almost all chronic conditions, Doyle accidentally stumbles over an alternative, which he dismisses instantly.

> Is it possible to provide sufficient home care services and supports that they [people with Alzheimer's disease] may be kept at home without, sooner or later, disrupting and almost destroying a family? Such a service would need to be very different from those we all know ... [necessitating] staff spending hours and hours a day with a patient (Doyle, 1990, p 6).

It is not the home care services and supports we all know that need to be different, but the institutional model that constrains home care services to be limited to what is seen currently. A system of appropriate home support services cannot be created while retaining a framework that centres care on the institution because, by definition, this framework must marginalise or make peripheral the home as a site of care.

Doyle seems to be unaware that in the disability field all around the world large numbers of people with support needs both similar to and in excess of the needs of people with dementia are managed all day, everyday, in normal homes by community living and support services, without the need for any institutions at all. The institutional model, by definition, implies it is the only way and that alternatives cannot possibly work unless, for example, as Doyle (1990, p 6) remarks, "unlimited resources" are made available. Alternatives to institutional care are made to seem unrealistic, inadequate, inferior, improper, idealistic, outrageously costly or naive.

However, Doyle (1990) is quick to acknowledge another effect, with relevance to what has always perpetuated the institutional model. "Public appreciation and support" for hospices would be "much less generous" and "professional rewards would be different, possibly less", if hospice care expanded into dementia care (Doyle, 1990, p 6). This is a blunt and perceptive admission of the realities of social devaluation. The devaluation deriving from idealised hospice care's fight against the unpalatable aspects of cancer and dying is institutionally very useful, for gaining generous public appreciation and support and for professional rewards. However, should palliative care become sullied with the devaluation attending care of the 'irrational elderly' then all these institutional privileges would be compromised. The devalued roles typically associated with dementia and with old age do not include the idealised, devalued role of 'holy innocent', except by virtue of old people being cast prematurely into the dying role itself, whereas in palliative care this romantic idealisation of devalued (dying) people is pronounced and prescribed. As a result, caring for older people who are 'losing their minds' is seen as far less special, rewarding and intimate than caring for people who are dying heroically, and are 'very close' or 'special' to God. If contaminated by the devalued roles associated with dementia and psychiatric conditions, the idealisation of people who are dying becomes much less useful for bestowing professional rewards, generating social approval and the whole array of institutional benefits enjoyed by palliative care. Seale (1998) also notes the lack of fit between the heroic revivalist discourse and modern ideas about older people.

'Complex need' and 'service gap' are two sides of the one coin. Every service has gaps. The term 'gap in the system' itself implies the current system can and should fill these gaps, when in fact these gaps are exclusions by the system, an inevitable outcome of the way the system is organised, as Strauss (1994) understands. People who fall through the gaps have, by definition, 'complex' or 'specialised' needs. All-encompassing hospices may try to solve the problem of gaps by maintaining, for example, an open door admission policy. In that case, the problem then is not that no service is available but that the service that is available is inadequate, inappropriate, inexpert and probably quite harmful. This occurs because the service available does not have adequate knowledge or expertise concerning the 'complex' need. 'High support needs' are liable to be deindividualised, given low priority or seen as equivalent to the needs of larger or traditional groups.

All-embracing institutions and their culture exclude people with 'complex' needs, either by not being able to provide adequate service, as in the case of the non-cancer illnesses generally, or, as in the following example, by refusing to provide any service at all. Gordon (1984) stresses the contradiction between the hospice principle that people must understand the nature of the referral to hospice and the admission of people with intellectual disabilities to hospice care. She states that "most [US] hospices interpret this [inability to understand the meaning of referral to hospice] to mean that dying persons who are mentally retarded are unsuitable candidates for hospice care" (Gordon, 1984, pp 165-6). To reiterate, this eventuality is not due to any complexity of people's needs but due to the way the institutional model is organised.

Complexity of need is relative to what the service provider provides. Non-traditional, complex or high support needs should be understood as exclusions by the culture and organisation of the service rather than the decontextualised, clinical view that sees such needs as objective facts displayed by individuals or groups. The 'complexity' of the needs of people with an intellectual disability who are dying is determined by a specialised service system whose organisation excludes this particular specialisation. People with an intellectual disability who are dying have 'complex' needs relative to an intellectual disability service provider because they are dying, and 'complex' needs relative to a palliative care provider because they have an intellectual disability. The institutional model cannot resolve its exclusions except by the ad hoc means of ever-increasing specialisation and institutionalisation, which itself further creates and intensifies the problems of exclusion.

Deindividualise and individualise care paradox

This paradox indicates that institutional approaches standardise or deindividualise care while aiming to individualise care. The prevailing view of palliative care is that it is "a medico–nursing set of services" (Kellehear, 1998, p 3). An institutional model, therefore, fits well prevailing ideas about palliative care. On the other hand, social models, such as health promotion, expand the sphere of concern beyond clinical processes to include the social context of the individual. For example, health-promoting palliative care seeks "a genuine social foundation for the idea of informed consent" or seeks to alter "community attitudes" regarding "the negative imagery and discriminating behaviour from others [which] the social realities of ... anything associated with death" evokes (Kellehear, 1998, pp 5-6).

Institutional models especially are locked into the reproduction of their prevailing mode of care. Just as acute hospitals must, by definition, 'diagnose-treat-cure', so hospices must, by definition, provide the nursing/medical services generally understood to be hospice care. The prevailing conceptualisation of palliative care is medical with religio-charitable overtones. The power of the service user to refuse, and the professional to not provide, this prevailing mode of care is very limited. Both staff and users must work within the various prescriptions or demands of this prevailing mode, even when basic rights of the user are denied or diminished by this prevailing mode of care.

A curious illustration of this denial is given by Saunders (1977), apparently as an instance of St Christopher's Hospice assisting people to protect their right to privacy. People who are dying are told this "rule": "'if you don't feel like talking with a stranger shut your eyes and pretend you're asleep'" (Saunders, 1977, p 172). The research and teaching imperatives of the hospice demand this denial of privacy. Although Saunders (1977, p 172) does institute some policy adjustments such as denying "visiting groups" access "to a ward or bay for a season" to try to moderate intrusions on residents' privacy, the hospice's research and teaching agenda, as well as the need to promote it as an open intimate community, require that the residents' right to privacy is compromised. By abrogating its primary responsibility to do no harm to the user, the hospice can only invent strange adaptations or institutional simulations of privacy. By reducing the only sure protection of people's right to privacy to a childish game, the hospice infantilises people, trivialising their privacy and the dignity it bestows. Asking people to pretend to be asleep in order to have privacy is an example of the type of devaluation called "life wasting" by Wolfensberger (1998, p 21). No such rule would ever be needed in a person's home, but the more complex conditions of the institution cause numerous weird individual and organisational adaptations because institutions cannot be what everyone thinks they are – the ultimate and total answer. Trying to individualise care so as to respect each person's privacy is impossible in any institution because policy can only refer to residents as a group of one sort or another, not as individuals. A privacy, or other, policy that is believed to be able to respect each individual's wishes at each moment is no longer a policy. Actually, it would be an organisational fiction, a delusion of institutional forms of management.

The right to privacy is not the only right denied or compromised by the prevailing concept of palliative care. For example, people do not have the same power to refuse treatment or control pain relief in hospice as they do at home, nor the same power to terminate contact, to complain, to determine appointment times or times of washing, recreation and the routines of living, nor the same power to have preferences met, to resist participating in teaching or research nor the same power to take risks.

SRV theory stresses 'the dignity of risk' (Perske, 1972). As Perske (1972, p 199) states: "the (real) world in which we live is not always safe, secure and predictable". By creating minimal risk, protective environments and activities, the dignity attaching to the risks involved in living is denied. A hospice cannot allow a person to take the same risks that he/she may take at home where risk taking is an entirely private matter, if only because of the hospice's duty of care and the risks to other residents. Risk taking has to be negotiated and deindividualised, rather than remaining a private decision on the part of the user system.

Residents of hospices and institutions will choose to try to fit into routines of every sort because they feel grateful and want to help, and because ultimately they know they have no choice. Small and Rhodes (2000, p 74) note that "the opportunity to leave a service or change to an alternative provider", called respectively "exit" and "redress" by Small and Rhodes (2000, p 74), is often specified as a prerequisite for meaningful choice. Even though there is virtually no opportunity to 'exit' and 'redress' in institutional care, institutional models still claim they both allow individual choice and offer high levels of accountability. The irony is that every time a person's rights or wishes are respected in institutional care, the person will feel grateful. People have to be grateful for every trivial personal choice that the institution respects when it is the institution that has already disallowed the basis for all meaningful choice, that is, disallowed the opportunity to 'exit' and to 'redress'. The compliance intrinsic to the medical and religious models compounds these kinds of problems concerning the denial of dignity, autonomy and choice under the institutional model. This intrinsic compliance is illustrated by Corley and Goren (1998, p 105), who stress the lack in nurses "of ethical consciousness of their use of coercive intervention and stigmatising of patients". Coercion is also discussed a little by Small and Rhodes (2000). Randall and Downie (1999) also discuss acquiescence, which is driven by the power inequality between service user and practitioner.

Depersonalise and personalise care paradox

This paradox indicates that institutional approaches depersonalise care while aiming to personalise care. Besides the depersonalisation caused by deindividualisation of service user needs, under institutional models authority and accountability become impersonal. Institutional models inherit an authority, status and respectability that is difficult to question, especially since it arises from no identifiable or accessible source. Communication channels become bureaucratised, complex and unclear.

The assessment of quality is constrained within the parameters of the 'benevolent institution myth' (Harris, 1995) and the prevailing conception of care. Criticism from alternative perspectives has marginal relevance or no meaning at all within these parameters. Quality assurance and accountability processes become institutional defences or self-congratulatory rites with little impact on the lives of people receiving care. Citing Argyris (1985), Corley and Goren (1998, p 110) emphasise that "organisations develop defensive routines that insulate their operative assumptions and mental models from scrutiny".

Personalisation of care involves the entire context of a service.

Personalised care begins with personalising access. For example, accessing home care services from a local, community-based palliative care service in a typical dwelling for the area without inpatient beds is very different from accessing home care through 'exactly the same' service provided from a more distant, large inpatient hospice or hospital.

Complicate and simplify conditions paradox

This paradox indicates that institutional approaches make conditions more complex while aiming to simplify conditions. 'Complex' symptoms or conditions in the home are supposedly relatively simple from the institution's perspective, since it is designed to control severe conditions and multiple contingencies. However, the setting itself imposes many new, complex conditions. For example, residents must watch and listen to other people suffer and die and their families grieve, just as the residents themselves grieve. In turn, those residents themselves will suffer and die, and their families grieve. And these people will then be watched and listened to by other residents and their families. Grouping people together places an enormous range of demands on them that would not exist if they were living at home, such as learning to navigate a new and busier terrain and learning to conduct very intimate times in relationships in a relatively public place. The report of a Mr Holden in O'Gorman and O'Brien (1990, p 44) is an example of this latter demand.

In institutional care, the intensification of experience alone that is imposed by institutional models must have many significant effects. Therefore, more importantly, none of these effects can be role valorising since they are achieved by a devalued means that requires as a precondition the loss of many roles. From an SRV-based perspective then, all these effects can only have a net, devaluing impact, no matter how beneficial the outcome might seem. That some effects might be considered positive, from certain clinical, interpersonal, individualistic or other viewpoints, demonstrates that devaluation is not understood and its effects ignored and hidden by processes based on these views. All such effects, when they occur in a hyper-intense environment for group dying, perpetuate death and dying as something outside ordinary ways of living. This is not to say that caring intentions or individual effects are necessarily made false by overarching devaluation, but rather that if we are unconscious of this devaluation, then caring intentions may be perceived as less-than-caring, unintentional harm may be done to a person and individual effects may not be what they seem.

As Connor (1998, p 145) states: "Anything that can be done in the hospital for a hospice patient can be done in the home as well". Everything that can be provided in a hospice, except group dying, can be replicated in the home. However, according to hospice philosophy, since the type of care not the setting is the critical element in defining hospice, it seems it cannot be group dying *itself* that causes the transformations reported as typical by Saunders (1977). If the hospice philosophy is correct, then hospices are not necessary in order for the transformations reportedly witnessed in hospices to occur. Hospice philosophy itself, therefore, appears to imply that the extraordinary personal benefits to people who are dying reportedly witnessed in hospices are no grounds for the existence of hospices. In other words, even if great things happen in hospices as people say, this anecdotal evidence, or any other evidence of consumer or public satisfaction, does not mean we need or should have hospices.

Part Three
Reconceptualising palliative care

SIX

An ideal palliative care model

Introduction

SRV's most significant impact occurs in the field of intellectual disability. The fundamental changes in this field since the 1960s reveal those key elements that need to shift in service systems in order to begin to remediate social devaluation. Central to restructuring these service systems is the conviction that institutional models are intrinsically flawed and unnecessary for classes at risk of social devaluation. The aim of this chapter is to envisage an ideal palliative care system by applying the key elements of SRV-based systems to the palliative care context.

This chapter argues that service systems can evolve beyond the institutional model to a dispersed services model. In the intellectual disability sector, SRV-based models have made substantial progress toward a dispersed, non-institutional service system. Following the same route, the first step required is to gradually close all palliative care institutions, replacing them with non-institutional or, at least, quasi-institutional alternatives. The second step required is to disperse the services delivered by palliative care organisations. All services should be dispersed among generic providers whose clientele mostly include people who are not similarly devalued, that is, people who are not dying. Case management should be separated from direct care to work against the concentration of services within one organisation. Specialist palliative care professionals should retain the case management role or its recently developed, more individualised, user-oriented forms, such as service broker.

Beginning with a discussion of the evolution of systems beyond institutional models, this chapter then looks at how a dispersion of service provision allows institutions to be closed. After examining the feasibility and effectiveness of non-institutional models of care, the chapter gives a description of the closure of a disability institution, a significant proportion of whose residents require palliative care. The chapter concludes by outlining a reconfiguration of case management that can work towards a dispersion of service provision.

Beyond institutional models

The intellectual disability services system has been reinvented to respond to the ethical demand to close all institutions. This evolutionary process is continuing. Although far from perfect, intellectual disability service systems in various countries have operated for a couple of decades in broad terms, without the need for any significant institutional expression except the small group home.

Deinstitutionalisation does not simply involve the closure of institutions. Deinstitutionalisation also involves the simultaneous development of a range of support systems to replace and extend in a more appropriate way the services provided in institutions. To try to allow a staged reintroduction to community living, a series of supported living options has been developed in the intellectual disability sector to give people time to develop competencies in living skills. Taylor's (2005) critique of this 'least restrictive environment' approach in intellectual disability services is a valuable guide to understanding the logic behind the structures of human service systems and also elucidates the critical flaw of this approach.

People's lives tend to get stalled, always being prepared but never being deemed by services to be ready for valued living. Staged reintroduction allows service system agenda to dominate. The demand that people must endlessly prove their readiness frustrates the urgent needs and dreams of people with an intellectual disability to begin to live a valued life in their own home. However, the 'least restrictive environment' approach does allow time for community supports to develop and adjust to the absence of institutions.

In the palliative care system, a hospice house with eight beds, for example, is a less restrictive environment than a larger hospice. With developments such as day care centres and palliative care units in hospitals, a number of additional environments represent further elements in the range between least and most restrictive environment. While institutions exist, the service system functions, in effect, as a feeder system for the most restrictive environment, the institution, which represents the end of the line. Institutions in this system are not disinterested parties and, therefore, institutional agenda as well as individual needs drive this movement toward the most restrictive environment.

Sanderson et al (1997, pp 154-63) describe the evolution of service systems beyond institutional models. Sanderson et al (1997, pp 154-63) explain that as service systems respond to demands for care to become more individualised, the service system becomes more complex. The institutional model is an elementary organisational form, since its ideology, culture, processes and structures are all simple conceptually, rigidly determined and confined within fixed standardised parameters. The rudimentary simplicity of the institutional model explains some of its appeal to social planners, governments and communities. The institutional model makes a loud and authoritative pronouncement that the personal and social disruption caused by dying, for example, is under the maximum possible control, because the institution of care provides 'total care' in the most restrictive or all-embracing way.

As institutions close, the service system needs to respond to the particularity of people's individual contexts and support needs. The central focus then shifts toward designing systems that can facilitate an individualisation of support and the social inclusion of people with an intellectual disability, for example, into the valued living patterns of each of their particular communities. Services become dispersed and patterns of service utilisation more complex. As Sanderson et al (1997, p 155) note, a "set of dispersed services – hostels, group homes, day centres, community teams" replace the institutions of care. While these developments, except possibly community-based teams, are still devaluing since they are quasi-institutional, they do provide a range of less restrictive environments than large institutions.

Sanderson et al (1997, p 154) refer to the 'dispersed services' model as the next step following the institutional model in organisational complexity. A case management approach to care, such as Provencal (1987), is used in which professionals work closely with people seeking support and their families to put together a package of services from various sources to meet individual requirements. This type of case management model facilitates the shift to dispersed services provided by a number of different agencies and avenues of support. This system became well developed in intellectual disability services in the US during the 1980s. While community-based palliative care teams are valuing to the extent that they support the maintenance of the role of home occupier, the structure of case management in palliative care does not promote a dispersion of service provision. In any case, without the preconditions to close institutions and break up services that provide the vast bulk of support, case management tends to revert to being just another way of moving people around the system, and eventually into institutions.

By the late 1980s and early 1990s, the evolution from dispersed services toward user-controlled systems began in earnest with the development of 'person-centred planning' (Sanderson et al, 1997). The lack of effectiveness of dispersed services and case management at facilitating anything more than a partial physical inclusion in communities created the impetus for the next developmental phase, called by Sanderson et al (1997, p 154) "person-centred services". Unless a formal commitment to SRV principles and understandings of devaluation is maintained, fashionable terms such as 'person-centred' can mean almost anything, and certainly can be used to justify devaluing practices that are the direct opposite of 'person-centred'.

A move away from case management to independent service brokerage and direct funding to people with a disability is also part of the current shift toward 'person-centred services' in which service users can have some say in how funding is spent. In this way there is a direct financial incentive for services to respond to the particular context of the individual. An example of direct payment policies, primarily but not only focusing on the disability sector, is the 1996 Community Care (Direct Payments) Act in the UK, discussed by Pridmore (2006). Lord and Hutchison (2003) investigate a number of individualised funding or support projects from the US, Canada and Australia.

The key elements, therefore, in shifting toward 'person-centred services' in palliative care, that is, toward a service and community system that can maintain people's valued roles and be fully responsive to each person's context are:

- to close palliative care institutions by using a dispersed services model; and
- to establish a dispersed services system via a new case management approach where one organisation does not provide the vast majority of support, and where service providers to any one person are independent of each other, exist within the community of the service user and do not solely service people who are dying.

Dispersed services

An ideal service, according to SRV principles, is one that centres care on the home (or other role-valorising environment) in an organisational sense, in order to defend the valued roles of people living in their homes and to improve the chance of people's needs and dreams taking precedence over the demands of the service system. To enable the transition from institutional care toward more home-like living, the key element in a 'least restrictive environment' approach has been the development of the community residential unit or small group home, a quasi-institutional setting.

People in institutions are relocated to community residential units in normal suburban houses that should be typical in every way for the area in which they are located. This interim solution allows the gradual closure of all institutions and facilitates, to some degree, the physical integration of people in a normal community. Houses with various levels of support are established, from independent living houses, with on-call support, to houses with 24 hours support each day. Even people with the highest support needs now live in community residences. People with the highest support needs benefit most from non-institutional care for a whole range of reasons, including that their care is the first to be compromised in institutions. Theoretically, the various levels of support in community residential units allow people a staged reintroduction to normal community living. However, because these units are structurally quasi-institutions and because of conceptual flaws in the underpinning 'least restrictive environment' model, institutional approaches persist in these units and social inclusion can remain minimal (Taylor, 2005). Nevertheless, a fundamental shift in the social imagery of people with an intellectual disability has been initiated since people with an intellectual disability have now become visible in communities with, for some, a visibility similar to that of valued people. Sanderson et al (1997) also discuss some of the problems of the staged supported living approach, which include that service dispersion can remain limited; social inclusion can remain negligible or non-existent; people have to change house as their independence grows; and professionals and house support staff can still dominate and govern care. Notwithstanding these reservations, in palliative care such a process on a very much smaller scale would allow a corresponding closure of all inpatient settings. However, there is minimal need for any such palliative care residential units in the longer term since the vast majority of people who are dying will be established in their homes in valued roles, as Chapter Four indicated.

The palliative care system can be seen as having made some moves toward a dispersed services model, principally by the provision of services in the home. For example, in terms of the scheme of Sanderson et al (1997, pp 154-63), a community-based palliative care team supporting people in their homes would be seen as a relatively dispersed service. Where people cannot move freely between such services because only one service is funded to serve one locale, or where a generic provider already provides similar services to people other than those who are dying, the degree of dispersion provided by such a palliative care team decreases. A hospice house of the US type would be seen as a mini-hospice, an institution or quasi-institution, to some extent a dispersed service relative to the larger hospices. The closer a hospice house is to a regular neighbourhood home, indistinguishable from other homes, the closer the hospice house comes to a dispersed service.

A development mentioned with reference to the US context by Schmoll and Dixon (1996, p 59) is AIDS-specific residences that are "owned and operated by hospices or they may be community based homes". As an example, the Connecticut Hospice cottage hospice, established in 1988, which is a "five bed house for the indigent, terminally ill [who have no home or no one to care for them at home]", soon began to focus on AIDS (Miller and Abbott, 1991, p 157). This house has some highly devaluing attributes because it segregates people with AIDS and is built adjacent to the Connecticut Hospice inpatient building. However, hospice houses do point to a tendency, at least in the US, toward the community residential unit innovation of the disability services sector. These units originated in intellectual disability services around the same time as related housing innovations in psychiatry were taking place under the influence of the anti-psychiatry movement, notably Laing (1965).

The popularity of hospice houses in the US may reflect a lingering attachment to the belief that the best site of death is the private home. The smallest hospice houses of 4-6 beds may particularly reflect this belief. However, the early drive in palliative care to assert the superiority of dying at home over institutional sites of death seems to have dissipated considerably into an acceptance of the rectitude of institutional management. This drive may still exist, however, by virtue of palliative care's romantic idealisation of people who are dying, and attendant romantic ideas about the naturalness of home death noted by Clark and Seymour (1999, p 22). This drive should not be confused with the present work that appeals to a rational basis for the intrinsic superiority of home death rather than to its romantic appeal. Nevertheless, in the healthcare system generally the shift away from institutional models appears to have some momentum. Some authors such as Newell (1996, p 228) believe the new (US) healthcare system based on nursing case management (or managed care) will continue to shift the focus from the hospital to the home. Many authors (for example, Blouin et al, 1996, p 178; Newell, 1996, p 228, p 231; More and Mandell, 1997, p 134) confirm indications toward the home becoming a focus of care. Ritter-Teitel (1996, p 59) notes, however, that there is no agreement about the "future position of hospitals in integrated systems". Nevertheless, the patterns evolving both in managed and community care internationally appear to support the evidence from the intellectual disability sector that case management models of some sort are the most direct way to work toward more dispersed service models where the institution of care is not the centre of care.

Closure of institutions

Feasibility

SRV theory argues that institutions for chronic or disabling conditions are unnecessary and always an inappropriate way of caring. (Acute hospitals should be utilised when the need is one for which any valued person would routinely use an acute hospital.) The institutional model is not exclusively the province of institutions. Although institutions are the clearest and most extreme example of the institutional way of caring and its negative effects, this approach to care can exist in some form or other in any setting. As well as indicating that institutional approaches can be imposed on the home, More and Mandell's (1997, p 134) statement that with managed care "many times homes are transformed into 'minihospitals'" indicates that the home can be made into a substitute for the hospital. Saunders (1977, p 160) conceives of St Christopher's Hospice as "something between a hospital and the patient's own home". A home can, therefore, be turned into a mini-hospice, and whatever can be provided in a hospice must be able to be duplicated in the home, and much more readily so than when the home is turned into a mini-hospital. In any case, whatever the arguments may be that support the claim that institutions are necessary for chronic conditions, ageing or dying, the intellectual disability service system over the past 35 years has proven the feasibility and sustainability of closing institutions in an entire sector across a number of nations.

Outside the field of intellectual disability, New York State's programme known as the Nursing Home Without Walls (NHWW), legislated in 1977 (Miller and Lombardi, 1991), shares concerns about institutionalisation. "The goal of NHWW is to reduce the human and fiscal costs involved in institutionalizing chronically ill persons while increasing the quality of life for individuals" (Miller and Lombardi, 1991, p 138).

While Miller and Lombardi state that NHWW allows more appropriate use of institutional care for 'those who really need it', a notion rejected by SRV theory, the idea behind NHWW implies

NHWW-like approaches can and should replace institutional care. Doty (2000) notes several approaches besides NHWW that seek to shift the focus of chronic care away from institutions. Doty's (2000) examination of the US evidence regarding the cost-effectiveness of NHWW and other alternatives to institutional care examines whether replacing long-term institutional care is a feasible financial alternative. The economy of the 'economies of scale' argument has always been conditional on excluding huge amounts of unmet chronic need in the community and further screening out according to perceived social value. This argument has always served powerful vested interests and been used to silence alternative voices.

While issues concerning cost-effectiveness, such as those raised by Doty (2000), are still being explored, NHWW has proven outside the specific field of intellectual disability the practical point that home and community care can support people with very high support needs in their homes. Randall and Downie (1999, p 206) note that "regrets should not be expressed that he [any person] did not die at home unless the available services had not provided all the care they could", and these authors go on to restate a variant of the 'economies of scale' argument – that resources will always be limited and care must be provided within available resources. Such an analysis begs the question about which resources should be available and how they should be organised or utilised. While an institutional system dominates the landscape and a community-based system has to be built up, naturally the institutional system appears most cost-effective. This pretence of economy can then sideline the ethical imperative to address social devaluation, while community support alternatives are portrayed as unproven, simplistic and financially and clinically irresponsible.

As mentioned earlier, contrary to the ideal of NHWW, SRV theory challenges the idea that anyone needs institutional care and adds that those for whom it is claimed institutional care is absolutely essential are the very people who will benefit most from non-institutional care. Not only do the smallest improvements in care make the most difference for people with high support needs, but also it is they who suffer most from institutional care, especially via neglect and abuse. For example, people who are dying, comatose or have severe communication difficulties can be readily interpreted as unable to respond to staff and show gratitude for care, an implicit institutional demand that is still clearly evident in the types of patients nurses prefer, as Corley and Goren (1998) indicate. The level of interpersonal identification with people receiving support is a key determinant of the support provided. The severe devaluation of people with high support needs means that they would be very likely to receive a less than equitable distribution of whatever amount of support happens to be available.

The practical achievement of NHWW with those with high support needs is impressive. Of NHWW patients, 46% live alone (Miller and Lombardi, 1991, p 142). Miller and Lombardi (1991, p 148) describe a couple in their early sixties – the wife with "multiple myeloma and bone tumours that caused spontaneous bone fractures", the husband with cancer of the colon requiring twice weekly chemotherapy. NHWW provided "personal care 12 hours a day, 7 days a week, and weekly nursing visits to monitor their physical condition. The NHWW nutritionist assisted with special diets, and a social worker provided supportive counselling". The wife also received physiotherapy and both had emergency response alarms. "This husband and wife were able to remain in their home together despite the seriousness of their illnesses, until they passed away within weeks of each other" (Miller and Lombardi, 1991, p 148).

NHWW was established to address

> the increased demand for long-term care, rising health costs, high incidence of premature/inappropriate institutional placements, and patient and family preference for care at home ... Nursing Home Without Walls having demonstrated its effectiveness in responding to these problems and trends, is now firmly established as an integral part of New York State's long-term care service (Miller and Lombardi, 1991, p 141).

In NHWW's development, those who see any alternative to institutional models of care as too idealistic, too expensive or simply unworkable came to the fore, as occurred with critics of the movement to close institutions in the intellectual disability services sector. The early development of NHWW was constrained by the "belief on the part of some local officials and providers that their communities 'already received an equivalent service' or the belief that the programme would 'only work in service-rich metropolitan areas'" (Miller and Lombardi, 1991, p 140). However, NHWW can demonstrate that "the program has enabled some persons already in an institution to return home, helped prevent at-risk community residents from further deterioration and eventual placement and afforded many the opportunity to die at home with dignity" (Miller and Lombardi, 1991, p 147). "Patient care costs under this program [NHWW] have consistently been about half the cost of comparable levels of institutional care. Since the program is a substitute for long-term facility care, the need for expensive construction is reduced" (Miller and Lombardi, 1991, p 139). Additionally, "to the extent that the program is able to improve patient functioning; help prevent accidents and deterioration; and minimise acute hospitalisation, emergency room use, and other high-cost medical care, its cost savings benefits are increased" (Miller and Lombardi, 1991, p 151).

The funding parameters of the healthcare system determine, to some degree, the extent of these observed and notional savings. As has been mentioned, the cost-effectiveness of NHWW, and other community care demonstration projects in the US, has been questioned and the level of savings reported by Miller and Lombardi (1991) appear not to be verified by further research examined by Doty (2000). Nevertheless, the principle that chronic and long-term care, including care for people who are dying, can be delivered in ways that foster a reduction in institutionalisation is demonstrated by NHWW, even if some kind of economic constraint on such a system were to prove necessary.

As well as services in the home similar to NHWW, some form of community residential unit may be useful temporarily in the palliative care system in the transition from institutional care, as has been mentioned. As interim measures, while the community-based sector adapts to the closure of institutions, such units could be used, for respite needs or, perhaps, for particular contingencies involving some non-cancer conditions. "Group residential housing arrangements" have been an "appealing option to [US] hospice providers" as an alternative to home and institutional settings such as inpatient and day care centres, and such homes have been evident especially in services to people with HIV/AIDS (Martin, 1991, p 38). Martin (1991) goes on to assert the cost-effectiveness of such a model, as does Tehan (1991, p 55). Again, services to a highly stigmatised group instinctively tend to point toward options that can provide some protection against devaluation.

Tehan (1991, pp 54-8) describes the operation of a hospice team working with a group home for people with HIV/AIDS and also the effectiveness of a related case management programme linking with a broad range of generic providers such as drug rehabilitation services. Tehan (1991) illustrates some of the types of roles required of a residential support team and a differentiation of roles between the hospice team and the residential support team of the AIDS organisation. This model, where the AIDS organisation is the primary provider and care manager, demonstrates the unconscious demand for dispersed services by people at high risk of devaluation. Palliative care is not being provided by the AIDS organisation, as would be the case under an institutional model, but by a 'generic' palliative care team, that is, relatively generic because it is servicing people other than those with HIV/AIDS.

Once institutional approaches are denied, there is an automatic tendency toward the utilisation of generic and dispersed services. Doty (2000) notes that some allowances for costs by US funding bodies for community-based models are below their nursing home equivalent because of the acknowledgement that under community-based models service users will still access generic services, such as their local doctor, whereas this cost needs to be included in the costs of the institutional nursing home. Doty (2000), and others such as Raetzman and Joseph (1999), note that the greatest challenge for non-institutional care from a cost perspective are those people with long-term, high-level needs. As noted, from an SRV-based perspective, it is improper either to target funding for non-institutional care at the population with less costly needs or to promote institutional care as the 'best' or 'only' option for people with the highest, that is, most costly, needs. In addition, the question of the cost of high support needs has limited relevance to people who are dying specifically, since relative to long-term chronic conditions these costs will be low due to the comparatively short periods of care.

There appears to be a connection between cost-effectiveness and community residential units. As has been mentioned, a whole range of notional cost savings appears to be associated with non-institutional alternatives such as NHWW. It seems counterintuitive to argue that, for an equivalent quality and quantity of care, institutional care is cheaper than community-based care, especially when in general there is some free carer input in the home and since most people do not need a home built because they already live in one. Nevertheless, after examining the research, Doty (2000) concludes that using group homes as part of a community-based system assists in achieving budgetary neutrality with respect to institutional alternatives. Doty's (2000) summary of cost-effectiveness research includes those, such as Kane et al (1998), who hold an optimistic view of the cost-effectiveness of community-based alternatives even under current US funding arrangements.

Clark and Seymour (1999, p 168) summarise the issues around cost specifically concerning palliative care in the following way:

> Bosanquet et al (1997) suggest little cross-comparative research has been conducted in the UK, although evidence

from the USA suggests that home-based care is more acceptable to both patients and carers, less costly and more equitably distributed than institutional hospice care. In the UK, the emphasis has been on ... evidence to improve care, rather than a critical analysis of the continued benefit of inpatient and hospice provision.

Justifications for institutions

No matter the proven financial feasibility, sustainability or effectiveness of alternatives to institutional care, people's belief that institutional care is the best and only option drives demand for it. When intellectual disability institutions were closed, people with a disability, families and professionals expressed many reasons to continue with institutions. However, several decades after the closure of almost all institutions the system, although by no means perfect, does in fact manage to support people with disabilities. People with a disability and their families generally have grasped with both hands the opportunity for non-institutional living. People with a disability and their families are generally no longer persuaded by the 'benevolent myth' perpetuated by institutions of care about their necessity and excellence. One powerful indicator of the success of SRV-based systems is that it would now seem almost preposterous, and certainly cruel, to suggest the system should return to mass institutionalisation.

Provencal (1987, p 5) summarises the most common justifications used to persuade people to opt for institutional care in the intellectual disability field:

- "He [the person with an intellectual disability] would be better off because he would be with his own kind."
- "She would be better off because the people who work in institutions are trained to look after people like her."
- "She would be better off because it is safe there."
- "He would be better off because you know that people will watch him."
- "They [staff] teach them [people with an intellectual disability] things that they would not be able to get if they stayed at home."
- "They have doctors right on the premises that can give whatever medical treatment might be needed."

Analogous arguments can be made to explain a preference for inpatient palliative care admission. The inpatient palliative care unit/hospice provides:

- the company and support of others who are dying ("be with his own kind");
- the 'special' knowledge, sensitivity and approach of staff ("people trained to look after people like her");
- the protective environment and therapeutic community ("safe there");
- the monitoring or surveillance ("people will watch him");
- the therapeutic community/institution that offers what the carer/ home cannot ("things they would not be able to get if they stayed at home"); and
- the ultimate reassurance through 'total' medical/nursing support ("doctors right on the premises").

Provencal (1987, pp 5-9) repudiates each of these arguments for institutional care. Provencal (1987) shows from his detailed description of a prime example of community-based service design how the fears entailed in such arguments are not substantiated in practice and how much improvement in people's lives is achievable under community-based models supporting SRV principles. The truth about institutional care, revealed in exposé after exposé, shows each of the claims to ultimate care by institutions to be unfounded. The superior quality of institutional care is a lie; the home can replicate the care in the institution. Total care is a lie – neglect is widespread. The protective environment is a lie; abuses of all sorts are rife in institutional care. The 'special' knowledge and sensitivity of staff is a lie; since often barely qualified people work in institutional care, since staff themselves are frequently the perpetrators of abuse and since, especially during the night, very inexperienced staff can be in control. And discussing the claim regarding surveillance in a little more detail, the 24-hour surveillance of institutions is a lie because people, especially those who are bed-ridden, can be ignored for many hours and response times to emergency calls can be long. A corresponding surveillance provided in the home would be one-to-one and, therefore, far more comprehensive, responsive and assured. Taylor (2005) disproves the claim to total or ultimate care by institutions, in respect of the intellectual disability sector. Citing several authors, Taylor (2005, p 98) states: "historically, of course, the most segregated settings provided the least intensive services". He continues that, with demands for institutions to increase service intensity to try to match the intensity of service able to be provided by community-based options, institutions as a result "capture a disproportionate share of expenditures on services" (Taylor, 2005, p 98).

The following discussion from Kellehear (1990) describes the social factors behind the institutionalisation of dying in the 20th century. Referring to Fulton (1972), Kellehear (1990, p 12) specifies the increasing representation of older people in the dying population as one such factor. Kellehear (1990, p 12) also specifies as factors "negative attitudes to intergenerational living and the extended separations of the chronically ill or dying [that] weaken social and emotional bonds". He continues by asserting that other broad social factors play a major role in discouraging people from choosing to die at home. These are:

(a) the growth of the view of death as a form of stigma, and
(b) the shift from acute to chronic types of illness and disablement, and
(c) radical decreases in exposure to death and dying and subsequent to this, of information about it. (Kellehear, 1990, p 12)

Regarding the factors dissuading older people from dying at home, Kellehear (1990, p 12), citing Kalish (1965, p 92), lists as factors: the "reversal of the parent/child relationship" involved in daughters/sons providing care for older parents, medical pressures (for example, concerning pain relief), psychological pressures (for example, being a burden), and financial pressures (for example, relinquishing carer income).

These factors given by Kellehear (1990) in the sociological background to the institutionalisation of dying are related to the social devaluation of people who are dying and their carers, with the exception of the population factor and, perhaps, the medical pressures. Addressing the social devaluation implications of the palliative care system will ameliorate, either directly or indirectly through resocialisation, almost all these barriers that discourage people from dying at home.

O'Connor (1995, p 54), citing Bowling (1983) and Mor and Hiris (1983), summarises the reasons people do not die at home: "most people want to die at home, but do not do so for social rather than medical reasons". For the vast majority, it is not the quality of medical, nursing or other clinical management that stops people from dying at home, but rather a range of social factors. Doyle (1990, p 3) stresses this same fact that, of itself, should demand a shift in palliative care's focus away from clinical to social care. For the vast majority, social factors not clinical concerns lead to institutionalisation. The palliative care literature focuses almost exclusively on improving clinical care, whether nursing/medical or psychosocial/spiritual clinical care, and tends to ignore how to affect change in the critical social factors that cause dying at home to break down.

The 'ultimate' care available in institutions is used to justify their existence. This view tends to argue that the quality of medical care in the home cannot be of an equivalent standard to that available from an inpatient setting. The more specialised palliative medicine becomes and the more colonised by the medical elite palliative care becomes, the more likely it is that this claim will be given even greater prominence in arguments that support the necessity of inpatient institutions. As has been noted, numerous authors acknowledge that the home can be made into a mini-hospital. Taylor (2005, p 98) states it this way: "any health-related, educational or habilitative service that can theoretically be provided in a segregated setting can be provided in an integrated setting".

However, the claim that a comparable quality of medical care available in an institutional setting cannot be provided in the home is actually a red herring for the vast majority of people who are dying. Since, as has been said, most people fail to die at home for "social rather than medical reasons" (O'Connor, 1995, p 54), the relative quality of medical (or other clinical) care in institutions compared to the home has little relevance to arguments about whether inpatient palliative care units or hospices are necessary. If these social factors are addressed, then dying at home should only break down in rare clinical circumstances and the need for specialised inpatient settings should virtually vanish. The chance that a person who is dying will die at home is "to a very great extent, [influenced by] the structure and functioning of the larger health-care system" (Germino, 1995, p 70). This influence includes being increased by the availability of palliative care (Germino, 1995, p 70, citing many authors), and decreased by the availability of inpatient hospice beds (Robbins, 1998). It would seem that the availability of palliative care home support promotes dying at home but that the existence of inpatient palliative care does the opposite. SRV theory understands such an eventuality to be a necessary effect of allowing the option of inpatient care. SRV theory also appreciates that the availability of adequate, appropriate in-home support is the critical element in avoiding institutionalisation due to the range of social factors mentioned.

Not surprisingly, the primary reason people do not die at home appears to be a lack of adequate, appropriate supports in the home, whether this is referred to as lack of informal carer(s) (Clark and Seymour, 1999, p 22, citing Seale, 1990; Clark and Seymour, 1999, p 97, citing Griffin, 1991), "lack of access to palliative care services" (Clark and Seymour, 1999, p 158, citing Hunt, 1997), "inadequate assessment of needs and planning" (Clark and Seymour, 1999, p 97, citing Griffin, 1991) or "community services ... insufficient to support a home death" (Small and Rhodes, 2000, p 74).

Other reasons include a "lack of support for informal carers" (Clark and Seymour, 1999, p 97, citing Griffin, 1991), which is also likely to affect the breakdown of "informal caring relationships in the last few days", noted by Small and Rhodes (2000, p 74). Neale (1993, p 59) reports a clear, positive impact for carers in many areas related to the present discussion from a community care management initiative increasing voluntary, neighbourhood supports to the home.

Another set of reasons can be referred to as "inadequate symptom (or pain) control in the community" (Small and Rhodes, 2000, p 74). Again, it seems reasonable to suggest that equivalent symptom management outcomes at home should be achievable if adequate, appropriate home support is made available.

Although it is not clear whether the following information is gathered from the study undertaken, Storey (2005, 'Why do patients not die in their Place of Choice?') reports that the reasons people do not die in their place of choice are: "inadequate assessment of patient needs and preferences; poor coordination of care; poor face to face communication; lack of information; lack of 24 hours a day D. [district] nursing; inadequate communication between day and out of hours medical services; inadequate equipment; aging carers or poor family support". This confirms the overwhelming role played by social and organisational factors that could be summarised as inadequate appropriate support at home, and also confirms the absence, or peripheral relevance, of clinical reasons for the inability to achieve the chosen site of death. Incidentally, Storey's (2005) report on the use of a 'preferred place of care' tool for 124 people shows that 93% died in their preferred place of care and, of this latter group, 86% died at home, which indicates the kinds of levels of home deaths that may be readily achievable by services such as the UK 'Hospice at Home' organisation, focusing on supporting the home as the centre of care.

Adequate appropriate home support is also clearly relevant to the broad social factors involved in people not dying at home, which are older age and low socioeconomic status, especially if living alone (Clark and Seymour, 1999; Small and Rhodes, 2000). "Cultural beliefs about the role of the family, and the value of hospital care versus home care" also play a role (Clark and Seymour, 1999, p 158, citing Hunt, 1997). SRV theory advises caution in any overriding of the culturally valued option regarding, for example, place of death and open/closed awareness context.

Small and Rhodes (2000, p 74) mention as another factor a personal sense of "greater security" in hospital and also raise the important questions about who actually does and should make the decision about where to die, which involves the right to decide to leave an institution. Randall and Downie (1999) discuss these issues at length, concluding that it is unethical for the user/carer/family to be the unit of care in palliative care. The imagined greater security in the hospital is part of the 'benevolent institution myth'. Impossible conflict of interest problems around how decisions to admit/discharge to/from institutional care are made are built into palliative care's present construction that considers the person/carer/family group as the unit of care. And to conclude the list of reasons that people do not die at home, Clark and Seymour (1999, p 158, citing Hunt, 1997) add "haematological malignancy" and "disease of rapid progression".

Except possibly for these last two factors and the cultural factors, increasing the intensity or variety of appropriate support to the home would seem to be able to have a very significant impact on all the specific reasons raised, including in providing adequate support for people with non-cancer conditions who are almost certain to receive palliative care from non-specialists according to Clark and Seymour (1999, p 159). Where the sense of greater security in hospital is an issue, providing higher than necessary levels of in-home support in the initial stages may remove this fear-based perception, as happens quite often already to allow service users and carers time to feel more secure at home. A 'whatever-it-takes' approach to supporting the home opens wide the as-yet-unknown possibilities for innovative adaptations, such as the one described by Neale (1993, pp 58-9) and numerous examples from the intellectual disability sector, such as Jay Nolan Community Services (JNCS, 2006).

Once the arguments concerning costs and the superior quality of institutional care compared to non-institutional alternatives are shown to be problematic, arguments about the necessity for institutional care tend to reduce to an appeal to the right of the individual to choose an institutional site of care or death. This argument seems to imply that if there were no inpatient palliative care facilities, then people would be denied any kind of institutional death. Even if the aged care sector were deinstitutionalised, people could still choose to die in hospital. If the implication is rather that non-palliative care specialised institutional dying would be inferior, then this only argues for an improvement in palliative care in other institutions.

Alternatives to the current institutional model are made to appear to be offering a choice between an all or nothing option. People come to believe that the choice is between, for example, inferior support in the home and parent–child role reversal or ultimate institutional care and no parent–child role reversal. If services like NHWW were taken for granted rather than institutional care, then this would change social ideas and expectations about what level of support is proper and possible in care at home. A recognition of the tragic realities of institutional living, its enforced loss of valued roles and its power to control and conform every aspect of a person's life, would mean that alternatives like NHWW would come to be seen as common sense and ethically essential.

Institutionalisation to avoid parent–child role reversal illustrates the kind of understandable trade-off between the role losses in institutional care compared with those entailed in parent–child role reversal. People tend to prefer to take the loss of roles forced by institutionalisation, since only the person receiving care suffers under this option, but both he/she and his/her children suffer under the parent–child role reversal option. Such a preference may also reflect socialisation into preferring the losses from being a 'sick person' to the loss of elements of the valued parenting role, because being sick is understood as a role that puts everyone at risk of devaluation. However, the reversal of the parent–child role implies inadequacies and dependencies that do not sit well with modern, individualistic social values.

The man in Germino (1995, p 71-2) for whom being at home while he is dying is "special" chooses ahead of time to be admitted to hospital for the last few days of his life "to protect his daughters and wife ... [so that] the memories of him dead would not destroy the joy of the home..." (Germino, 1995, p 72). Several options besides his institutionalisation are possible to address these concerns and reassure everyone. However, examples like this one cannot be used, as the 'right-to-choose-site-of-death' argument does, to claim that the system should be configured around allowing this choice to die in an institution. Such examples merely indicate that, even if a person persists with this choice under a dispersed service system and socialisation away from institutional dying, then a deinstitutionalised system should be flexible enough to cater for this choice in the ways described earlier. By continuing with an institutional system, the choice of the many who wish to die at home is denied. It is unjustifiable to continue with this system that denies the choice of the many because the choice of the few who wish to die in inpatient care may be denied under a deinstitutionalised system.

Closure of Xavier's Children's Hospital

The "transformation of Xavier's Children's Hospital [for children with medical difficulties and disabilities, and severe and multiple disabilities] to Xavier Children's Support Network" (Card, 1999, pp 50-61) brings together much of the discussion so far in this chapter. This example illustrates an institutional closure and the means to facilitate it that would be possible for almost any hospice or inpatient palliative care unit. The transformation was motivated by government pressure for the transition to community care required by legislation (Card, 1999), the federal 1991 Disability Services Act (Parliament of Australia, 1991), which is based on the principles of SRV (Ziegler, 1992, p 11). Notably the transformation prioritised the home as the focus of care using a "whatever it takes" approach (Card, 1999, p 59) to providing support to allow children to remain living at home. A key worker, from the specialist disability service, Xavier Children's Support Network, was used to access dispersed services under a case management approach. Xavier Children's Support Network gradually withdrew from providing the bulk of direct care, previously undertaken by the hospital, and integrated the people it served into a network of services and supports (Card, 1999, pp 51-2).

A comparison between quality of life before and after the closure of the institution noted that although the hospital had cared for the children "extremely well" (Card, 1999, p 57), a quantum leap in quality of life at home was witnessed, of a kind unattainable within the institution. "Children have blossomed since moving home and are very happy" (Card, 1999, p 57). The negative side to their deinstitutionalisation was that reports claimed that "some children's health may be compromised", which Card's article implies occurred because of a reduced quality of medical care. However, these same families still reported that the children's overall quality of life had improved. Card (1999) notes that this balancing of trade-offs in care is the parents' responsibility. Naturally the trade-offs in institutional care are significantly more widespread and profound than those under a supported living model. Under an SRV-based model, improvements to quality of medical care could be developed in response to such trade-offs by, for example, increasing nursing/medical support to the home. Medical care at home can be made to resemble medical care in an institution almost completely. However, quality of life in institutional care is necessarily of an entirely different order to the quality of life attainable at home, no matter how home-like the institutional environment may appear or how sensitive, open and compassionate the staff.

In any case, Card's (1999) article records only the transitional phase to explain the process of closing the institution. Although Card (1999) does not imply this, the parents' expectation of receiving the total care that institutions unjustifiably portray themselves as providing may be involved in parents reporting decreased health in some children. As a result of this ultimate care image of institutions, the fears of the families themselves concerning their ability to deliver some aspects of medical care may also be involved. Some extraneous factors seem all the more likely since the external evaluation conducted at the end of the transition period is not reported to have made recommendations to improve medical care (Card, 1999, p 59).

The resocialisation of parents away from institutional models is evident. Card (1999, p 57) contrasts the attitudes of 'old' parents of institutionalised children, who felt institutional care had been their only option, with those of the 'new' parents, whose children had only known the family support model. The 'old' parents, even when visiting regularly, had to relinquish responsibility to the institution. The 'new' parents want to "assume and maintain responsibility from the beginning and want support and assistance, but not [have] their decision-making power removed" (Card, 1999, p 59). While an institution, such as a hospice, may allow family some level of participation in care, the ultimate responsibility for care is relinquished and given over to the institution. This fundamental shift in power signifies the real action on which institutional care is predicated, the denial and ongoing erosion of the valued social roles of user/carer/family.

Perhaps the most eloquent testament to the nature of the new order of quality of life in non-institutional care comes from the children with communication difficulties from Xavier's Hospital. "Children unable to communicate their feelings were seen [following release from the hospital] to sleep better, to demonstrate less stress behaviour, to attempt communication with others, to eat better and all showed an increased positive response – they smiled and consistently responded to carers" (Card, 1999, p 53). When carers, staff, family and friends, service providers of all sorts, acquaintances and people in the street can live among and witness this kind of transformative change in people's lives, the community itself is changed and the impetus for community to act as an agent of change can take root. Instead of the despair caused to people who are dying and families/carers by admission to institutional care of one sort or another, and witnessed by the community as the wholesale uprooting of a local identity, a community including the person who is dying can begin again to share together the profound responsibility for the life, dying and death of its members.

The transformation of Xavier's Hospital teaches many important lessons with relevance to palliative care. Two of these lessons are the important role and nature of leadership in change and the way to stage the gradual process of closure and the dispersion of services. Card (1999, p 51) emphasises: "I was the first ever non-religious, non-medical Director". The de-emphasis of the nursing/medical and religious models at leadership levels is evident. A shift in power and culture at leadership level greatly assists in breaking out of the existing model of care. Without it, the model of care can remain locked within the existing paradigm, an institutional medical model with religious ethos, despite the patent advantages of a model based on supported living and social valuation. Xavier Hospital had remained locked in its institutional model despite even legislative pressure. Leadership had to be open to and placate the fears of all stakeholders regarding the workability at every level of the new model (Card, 1999, pp 52-3). Change was implemented only gradually.

The first step was that institutional respite services were scaled down by the provision of additional options such as a respite house, an adaptation of the idea of a community residential unit. Options for family support were then developed. One service that was integral to family support packages was palliative care, since approximately 10% of the 130 medically fragile children required palliative care. Card (1999, p 57) specifies that family-based palliative care replaced institutional palliative care for those children who were dying in the hospital and, although she does not specify clearly, it appears that the palliative care service was not one run by Xavier's Services for the children of Xavier's Services alone. If this was the case, utilising such a palliative care service represents a greater move toward a dispersed services model than if Xavier's staff provided the family-based palliative care after the institution was closed. Although it is again not clearly specified, medical and nursing services to deinstitutionalised children who were not dying would have presumably been provided by non-Xavier staff, perhaps from their parents' local GP or from a community nursing service. The key worker of Xavier Children's Support Network, in consultation with children and their families, would have developed an integrated package of care for each individual. The social devaluation of children with a disability is reduced by the use of any other service, such as the palliative care service or local medical clinic, which serves people other than children with a disability.

SRV theory accepts a gradual evolution of the service system toward more role-valorising approaches. Citing Provencal (1987), Rouget and Harris' (1994, p 14) rule is a general one even though they are referring to service user participation in intellectual disability services. When an ideal solution is not achieved, accept any improvement and begin again to seek change toward the ideal rather than becoming complacent or giving up. As an example of this principle, which Rouget and Harris (1994) refer to as 'purism versus complacency', if a simple SRV-based change is not achievable this lack of purism should not be over-emphasised and interfere with moving toward other SRV-based changes. In the case of Xavier Children's Support Network (Card, 1999), changing the name from that of a Catholic saint to moderate the religious identifications of care has not been achieved to date, presumably because the service is operated by the Franciscan Missionaries of Mary. Nevertheless, almost the entire service model has been transformed from a medical and religious model to one based on the principles of SRV through Card's leadership. A different leader might have tested his/her power or acceptance and sought first to change the name.

New case management approach

Organisational context

Greene (1992, p 11) notes that "case management has been a traditional part of social work since the days of Mary Richmond", that is, since the inception of US social work in the late 19th century. Clearly, community nursing, as Clark (1996, p 295) notes in respect of public health nursing in the 1900s in the US, and community medical care have always involved some degree of informal care coordination.

Lee et al (1998) suggest that one reason for the lack of clarity concerning case management definitions and practices in nursing is that nursing case management is "in its infancy". Various aspects of care coordination have a long history in social work education, as the list of US social work competencies in Hollis and Taylor (1951, pp 222-4) indicates. Rubin (1992, p 14) reports that, while there is no clear consensus about the discipline that provides the best preparation for case management, "social work, public health nursing, vocational rehabilitation and human services generalist practice" are those areas often considered to do so.

Although questioning the competence of nurses acting as case managers in areas other than acute care is justified, the relevance to the present discussion is that, even in social work literature with its long-standing focus on case management, a notion central to SRV theory has been almost entirely overlooked. Friesen and Briggs (1995, p 63) explain that case management has been conceptualised as an "independent variable" abstracted from its context, ignoring the "influence of the organisational and inter-organisational context on the way that case management services are or can be delivered". Friesen and Briggs (1995, p 64) specify developments in mental retardation and mental health in the 1960s as beginning formal policy initiatives in service coordination. Friesen and Briggs (1995, p 64) state they are interested in the contexts of organisations not only because they explain why organisations are the way they are, but because "structural and organisational dimensions [are] legitimate objects of intervention". SRV theory strongly supports this view. SRV theory also emphasises that, because service processes with individuals are constrained and conformed by structural and organisational dimensions, clinical processes, for example, are not able to be understood separately from structural and organisational dimensions. If these dimensions are not reformed as legitimate objects of intervention, individually focused processes necessarily perpetuate any tendencies toward social devaluation that there might be at the broader structural and organisational levels.

For example, people are routinely encouraged to bring a few items from home to make their hospice environment home-like. This intervention tries to compensate for the devaluation of institutionalisation by trying to imitate valued living at home. This individual level intervention is corrupted by the overarching negative influence of institutional care, an organisational level influence. Necessarily, as compromise solutions that do not challenge the underlying organisational dimensions of devaluation, 'solutions' like bringing in a few items from home devalue people in new ways. This adaptation, for example, tends to trivialise, or at least commodify, a person's life as something able to be encapsulated by a few precious items.

Unless such contradictions are seen as inherently imposed by the institutional setting and seen as valid objects of intervention, the new devaluation is 'normalised'. This is not to say we should not encourage people to bring items from home. On the contrary, probably people should be encouraged to bring in the kitchen sink as well, so as to stretch the compromise 'solutions' of the institutional model beyond the organisational comfort zone. Although this suggestion is not intended seriously, since it would place vulnerable people at greater risk, it does indicate a generalised approach. The practical possibilities in any such compromise 'solution' can be exaggerated to show up the inherent devaluing contradiction in the policy, process or principle. Exaggerated possibilities may be raised at a staff development session, for example, and used to explore where, how and why the service draws the line between reasonable and unreasonable options.

It is hard to know what Saunders (1977, p 168) means when she says: "the way a patient is welcomed [regarding clothes, possessions, idiosyncrasies] into the new life of a hospice can be a reaffirmation of his own home and community, even though he may never return to them". In any case, since the hospice community shares some social responsibility for the loss of a person's real community, actions to reaffirm what was lost could be seen as two-faced. The hospice community, in effect, imposes this loss, by utilising institutionalisation as a way of providing care and by not being prepared to do whatever it takes to resolve the social issues that predispose people to being institutionalised. Although bandaid 'solutions' are then applied to try to value the lost life, the hospice community, in effect, implies by the act of institutionalisation itself that, however valuable the lost life was, it was not valuable enough to warrant being preserved.

Saunders' statement also appears to imply that the extraordinary value of the new institutional life being entered into in a therapeutic community enables it to somehow compensate for this loss, which implication, of itself, devalues the person and his/her lost life. To effectively impose a loss as significant as that of a person's own home and numerous, attendant valued roles on a person who is dying seems unjustifiable. For palliative care, which has drawn much attention to the importance of grief and loss issues, imposing loss upon loss on a person who is dying can only be counterproductive, at best, in terms of dealing with grief and loss.

Seen in this light, when clients refer to being in hospice as having 'come to Heaven', as 'coming home' or as 'a home away from home', these sentiments should be understood in the context of an internalisation of devaluation. Subjective reports from people who are dying and carers about palliative care services must be interpreted within the framework of internalised devaluation. Kristiansen et al (1999, pp 420-3) describe three processes that make using subjective criteria of life or situation satisfaction problematic, especially for devalued people. If the likelihood of devaluation effects is acknowledged, then the meaning of subjective opinions can be evaluated more sensitively and such information be understood more objectively.

When a carer expresses delight with institutional hospice care and, at the same time, feels guilty about having admitted his/her spouse, which is very common, then the carer has a vested interest in seeing hospice care as exemplary in order to ease his/her guilt about the admission. The feared repercussions for his/her spouse in the hospice and the feared repercussions of the loss of home for the person who is dying are important incentives to see the hospice as a 'wonderful place'. If the client is an unwilling or begrudging admission, this effect is increased. Institutional culture says that, while this guilt is understandable, it is irrational or unjustified because 'you (the carer) did everything you could' or, because 'we (palliative care support) did everything we could'. Institutional culture will not even hint at validating the carer's instinctive knowledge that institutional care will deprive the person who is dying of so very much, not to mention avoiding any hint that there is almost always more support or different support that can be provided. However, institutional culture must validate the carer's assumption that all that could be done to keep the person at home was done because a central assumption of the existence of institutions is that the institution is always the 'more that can be done'.

The service system and the expectations that the dominant institutional culture engenders determine when the limit of possible supports in the home has been reached and on what basis this determination is made. Naturally, this determination can only be made in such a way as to ensure the survival, and so the dominance, of institutional care. Spending 90% of the last year at home does not conflict with the hospice since it only wants to deal with the last few weeks of 'terminal care' anyway. The hospice only has to act to protect its interests to ensure this situation continues. Without the hospice, and with a 'whatever it takes' approach to home support, these last few weeks could also be spent at home quite readily.

Almost without exception, there is more that can be done or something that can be done differently to improve support to a person or carer at home, although none of this is relevant to or appreciated by the institutional mindset. Although SRV strongly endorses seeking the service user system's opinions and perspectives, these views must be interpreted within the framework of social devaluation and its internalisation. That very little bad is said about hospice care and particularly about hospices themselves, especially by users and carers, tends to support rather than deny the reality of internalised devaluation, since necessarily much unconscious harm must be done in palliative care, as anywhere.

The individual level cannot be understood without the organisational. Since so much of medical/nursing, religious/spiritual and psychosocial intervention is clinical in palliative care and, therefore, generally unconscious of organisational and structural influences as a whole, the level of unconscious devaluation occurring via individual interventions is likely to be very high.

While SRV theory points to the often unconscious influence of organisational factors such as setting, staffing and image, Friesen and Briggs (1995, pp 64-7) point to functional biases behind the idea of case management. The conflict between rationing resources through denying services to those deemed ineligible, via screening processes and, at the same time, trying to provide quality care, underlies all case management. Friesen and Briggs also confirm "that the clinical background of service coordinators contributes to their tendency to overlook the impact of organisational structure on services" (Friesen and Briggs, 1995, p 66, citing Norman, 1985). Since palliative care structures nurses into the case management role, a significant lack of awareness of the devaluation from organisational and structural dimensions is to be expected.

The organisational structure of palliative care means that case managers can also provide direct care. If these two functions are confounded organisationally, what is the impact on the way service is provided? What is the impact on accountability of direct care, for example, if a person receives direct care from the same person who provides case management services?

This problem deriving from the organisational context of case management in palliative care is made more worrisome by the fact that the distinction between case management and direct care is not black and white, as Randall and Downie (1999) assert. For example, a palliative care nurse case manager when interviewing a person is likely to be engaged in taking a medical history or assessing certain aspects of physical functioning that could be considered direct care. Case management primarily concerns care assessment, review and coordination of a more encompassing nature than similar tasks at the direct care level. For example, palliative nursing direct care involves ongoing assessment of pain management day to day. However, ongoing assessment in palliative nursing case management might involve periodic monitoring of overall nursing management including pain management, both directly via user/carer contact and indirectly via direct care nurses, other service providers and the user's file. Providing a rationale to categorise and separate these roles appropriately to avoid devaluing effects is the key to unravelling the complexity of the current internal organisational structure of palliative care services.

To generate a dispersed services model, case management should be structurally separated from and organisationally independent of direct care. Distinct role definitions for each member in the palliative care team should reflect this separation of case management from direct care. Role definitions should ideally reflect the utilisation of dispersed services for direct care rather than structuring the specialised palliative care team to act in direct care roles.

Separating case management from direct care

Muddy terminology regarding case management means that wrong understandings about how case management operates or what constitutes case management are widespread, particularly among nursing/medical personnel where it is a relatively recent development formally. SRV-based models demand an 'interagency' case management model, using Early and Poertner's (1995) scheme. A dispersed service model of palliative care would increase the involvement of generic service providers, shifting from what is now called an interdisciplinary team case management model in palliative care to an interagency model. At present, the palliative care team predominantly provides the vast bulk of direct care, although in some cases various limited components of care are dispersed to other agencies, such as to a GP, creating the beginnings of an interagency team on top of the interdisciplinary one. Except for hospital ward model assumptions, there are no criteria in palliative care to determine the services that should be dispersed, and those that should be provided directly by the interdisciplinary team. Except for hospital ward model assumptions, there are no criteria to determine the services that should be provided by specialist palliative care agencies and those that should be provided by generic agencies.

While this book is not the place to detail such SRV-derived guidelines, in order to generate dispersed services, specialist palliative care services/professionals should retain case management roles, including some direct care assessment role, and generic providers should deliver direct care. As an illustration, Randall and Downie (1999) maintain correctly that nurses should not be structured into [nor therefore perform] an advocacy role in palliative care for the reason mentioned in Chapter Five. In relation to community care in general,

Neale (1993) discusses changes to care management policy in the UK that affirm the principle of separating case management from direct care. Citing the House of Commons Social Services Committee (1990), Neale (1993, p 58) states:"the idea of care managers being independent of service providers, thus separating the interests of users and providers, and leaving the care manager untrammelled by organisational constraints, has been strongly advocated". In Australia, this separation of interests is also favoured regarding case management for people with a disability (Office of the Public Advocate and Headway, 1992).

The first step to creating a dispersed service network is to distinguish and separate case management from direct care. The palliative care service must retain some involvement in case management functions, which necessarily will involve some basic level of direct care as has been discussed, so that accountability of other providers and standard of care can be assured. Specialist palliative care services retain the specialised knowledge about palliative care. Case management is one potent way this knowledge becomes disseminated to generic providers. Once case management and direct care roles are distinguished by defining them strictly, generic providers can assume responsibility for direct care. If there are two tiers of expertise in direct care, then it is certain that over time those at risk of social devaluation will tend to receive the less expert level of care, as existing inequalities in access to palliative care may already indicate. Those who are more socially valued will tend to receive the care of specialists. Two tiers of expertise necessitate determinations about who is more or less deserving. Such determinations express the relative social value of various groups, and are also system–driven as much as needs-driven.

Establishing the separation of case management and direct care does not have to occur all at once. Gradual shifts toward a dispersed services model can be implemented even while a specialist palliative care service continues to provide all direct nursing care, for example. Whatever else is needed – medical services, massage, support groups, grief/loss education, relaxation, reading material, social events/lunches, religious/spiritual services, hairdressing, meditation, financial advice, legal advice, funeral advice, complementary therapy, music therapy, naturopathy, recreation, entertainment, and so on – the palliative care service should work to establish connections between relevant generic services and the person who is dying.

However, the current assumptions and interpretations of the provision of holistic care imply that a palliative care service should deliver most, if not all, of the elements of holistic care. This rule is based on the service's increased palliative care expertise and the unconscious importation of assumptions of the institutional medical model. In this way, palliative care services come to believe teams should consist of a spread of practitioners that can cover the entire range of the more common holistic needs.

Under the current palliative care structure, holistic care is nominal or marginal because of the medicalisation of case management. Because nurses drive case management referral within the team, the psychosocial/spiritual disciplines become marginal. These disciplines are reliant on nurses' assessments of psychosocial/spiritual need. However, under a dispersed services model, case management remains with a specialised palliative care service, or with generic case managers in collaboration with specialist services, depending on how a person enters the system. Under this new role for specialist services, opportunities to develop new case management structures arise in which neither the nursing/medical nor psychosocial/spiritual stream is accentuated or marginalised. The holistic definition of palliative care can then be operationalised by a more holistic case management structure. To move toward these new structures even under existing systems, case management staff should be separated organisationally from direct care staff, even though all staff might still remain within the one palliative care service that provides the vast bulk of support.

The details of how to restructure case management and direct care functions are beyond the focus of this book. However, three general principles are involved. First, reduce the nursing dominance of case management structures by, for example, creating two-person mini-case management teams comprising a medical/nursing stream specialist and a psychosocial/spiritual stream specialist, both of whom directly assess every person automatically. Second, separate case management and direct care organisationally, either by creating a distinct independent organisation, or mini-teams, as mentioned, or a case management team and a direct care team without any crossover of personnel. Third, exclude direct care nurses from case management immediately. Serious conflict of interest issues and the attendant dangers for service users intersect with the most urgent and critical clinical issue. In palliative care nursing there is an inappropriate yet inescapable and automatic transfer of nursing/medical authority into psychosocial/spiritual domains when the nurse acts in any but the most rudimentary fashion to provide psychosocial/spiritual support. This transfer of authority, trust and compliance is a necessary effect of the procedural touch fundamental to the nursing role. Establishing trust and authority via touch is unavoidable and necessary for nursing care. However, it is unethical that this authority and trust transfer, as they must automatically, when the nurse works outside the nursing domain, which is a structural demand in palliative care. Since the complexities of case management assessments routinely structure nurses to work in highly technical areas of the psychosocial/spiritual domain, such work is impossibly corrupted by the effects of procedural touch.

Strauss (1994) supports fundamental structural change to the US healthcare system because of the inadequacy of its chronic care systems and the inequity of care provision. Strauss (1994) stresses that the organisational focus on acute care, the hospital and clinic must change and will be forced to change by the "expected increase of *long*-end-of-life existence on the edge, more or less, of death. The issues are quite obviously moral at core, and the death and dying movement has taught us also that the issues are also psychological and medical/psychological. But they are also *organizational*" (Strauss, 1994, p 28; original emphasis). Strauss understands that the individual and organisational levels interpenetrate. Without organisational change, attitudinal change can be hollow, impotent or simply continue to perpetuate the social devaluation deriving from organisational levels.

SEVEN

Reconceptualising death

Introduction

The contradiction that palliative care devalues people who are dying while aiming to value them asks many questions of palliative care. Since palliative care seeks to change society's attitudes to death and dying, this contradiction must have some reflection in palliative care's understanding of death. This book argues that this contradiction shows a deep confusion about devaluation and its processes. Something in palliative care's understanding of death as it relates to devaluation must, therefore, intersect with this contradiction and help sustain it.

This chapter seeks to explore this connection with palliative care's conceptualisation of death that, naturally, reflects rather than challenges modern values and understandings of death. The discussion analyses the romantic idealisation of the compassionate ethos of the public health approach of Kellehear (2005a) and, by implication, the romantic idealisation of the religious ethos of palliative care. Understanding the conceptualisation of death behind this idealisation makes clear the costs, with respect to the meaning of death, of universalising death and loss. Key nuances arising from the insights of SRV theory enable this monolithic and universalistic idea of death to be disassembled. In this process, death is revealed to be a triune symbol that explains the appeal of the romanticisation of death, refines the understanding of death and expands the symbolic force and meaning of death. The chapter begins by setting the groundwork for exploring the three faces of death. Using a ground breaking and unifying concept from Wolfensberger (1992a) to contextualise the idea of death, the discussion then turns to deriving the triune face of death.

Making and unmaking death

It is necessary to make a preliminary qualification. Any reconceptualisation of death concerns a wide range of academic disciplines. The following explorations use the restricted assumptions and theoretical positions already established in earlier chapters without reference to the bodies of literature from other relevant fields. This is not meant to dismiss or ignore the work of others but to try to give form to these indications in a way that is relatively accessible, that does not overlay the weight of religious and philosophical discourse in particular, and that is directly and specifically relevant to palliative care's current conceptualisation of death.

The previous chapters indicate how palliative care devalues people who are dying, while aiming to value them. Part of Chapter Four aimed to show how the recent public health approaches of Kellehear (2005a) also, for the most part, tend to fall victim to this same fate. Palliative care's philosophical basis could serve as a vehicle for the following analysis. However, the current clinical emphasis of palliative care means that it is critically disengaged, in general terms, from the concerns that most affect it. Palliative care's conceptualisation of death is murky, mostly implicit and not well explicated, except in so far as it imports the traditional Christian meaning of death.

On the other hand, much more suited for this discussion's purpose is the pioneering work of Kellehear (1999, 2005a) that explores broader social horizons for palliative and end-of-life care and also suggests communities develop their own social capital to respond to the questions put by death and loss. In Kellehear's (2005a) work, the reach of the explicit conceptualisation of death and loss, the engagement with sociological literature and the broad social understanding of end-of-life care exceeds much palliative care discourse. Kellehear's (2005a) critique of normalisation, social justice and difference-based approaches, as well as his emphasis that death and loss are socially and individually instructive, bring to light aspects of palliative care's notion of death that are yet to find clear expression in the more conventional palliative care literature. For these reasons, the following analysis uses the 'compassionate cities' (Kellehear, 2005a) approach as the vehicle for the development of an expanded conceptualisation of death that is directly relevant to both 'compassionate cities' and palliative care. This discussion does not seek to minimise the importance of Kellehear's (1999, 2005a) work but rather seeks to use it as a vehicle to redefine the meaning of death in general, with specific relevance to palliative and end-of-life care.

Earlier chapters show that, for the most part, both palliative care and Kellehear's (2005a, p 34; original emphasis) approaches understand death and loss as "*universal and normative* experiences". Furthermore, both approaches believe that death subsumes loss categorically, that is, that every loss is a symbol or prefiguration of death, a mini-death so to speak. Every loss, grief and suffering is an encounter with ever-present death, who is all at once stalker, companion and wise counsel. These beliefs drive both approaches to aim to make death, dying and loss normal, valued parts of life, integrated into all aspects of society. However, both approaches aim to achieve this reintegration of death into everyday living patterns in ways that necessarily perpetuate the devaluation of people who are dying, although palliative care does so much more directly than Kellehear's (1999, 2005a) approach.

Both approaches use a romantic idealisation of death to try to achieve this reintegration or revaluation of death. The analysis undertaken shortly reveals the necessity of some form of idealisation of death, although not because of the need to cloak its sinister and aggressive side. At the same time, the analysis shows that the romantic idealisation in both approaches is based on reductive assumptions about the meaning of death. Both approaches see clearly that death and dying are devalued by society, but seem to confound statistical and social normativity concerning death and loss. Nevertheless, both approaches seek to reinstate death in its age-old role of wise counsel and ever-present shadowy companion. Under a universalising notion of death, its sinister associations from its ever-present sense of threat and warning, for example, can only be positively reframed through some sort of romanticisation of the scary side of death. Sinister associations of death, as a universal, have to be seen as beneficial, at least in the end, for both individual and society. The standard and very old romantic means, which both approaches have borrowed, is to conceive of death as wise counsel, or symbol of conscience, teaching hard, age-old lessons that only death can deliver or that death delivers best.

Palliative care's romantic idealisation of death is a religio-medical one invoking the goodness of religion and the "love in action" (Bradshaw, 1996, p 412) ethos. Religious idealisation in palliative care's view of death implies that, at least, people are reassured that once dead they have the promise of peace. To cover all contingencies, palliative care's romanticisation adds the goodness of medicine, and its implied indefinite progress, to convey that the unpleasant or painful side of dying is increasingly manageable. If this happens not to be so in a specific case, the love and companionship of palliative care personnel prior to death are there to reflect or mediate the promised peace. Kellehear's (2005a) romantic idealisation is a quasi-religious one, invoking the absolute good of compassion and the universality and statistical normativity, or commonality, of loss and death. For Kellehear (2005a) death, in its actual form, and loss, one of death's symbolic forms, can teach society compassion and, therefore, death and loss can be used by various social processes to encourage the development of compassionate communities.

Kellehear (2005a) sees a number of problems with focusing on death, dying and loss as a difference, or devalued characteristic, rather than as a common experience shared by us all. Understanding that a focus on the difference of death confirms, in some abstract sense, the truth of the devalued attribution, Kellehear (2005a) supports a universalising of death and loss as shared human commonalities, as does palliative care less explicitly. And this universalising is the root of the problem with the romantic idealisations of both approaches. The universalisation of death embraces all death, as it does all loss. As a result, critical qualitative nuances in the meaning of death are denied, overlooked or flattened out. Death and loss become a homogeneous qualitative mass fundamentally only varying in a quantitative way. Under this view, the loss of a pet, a job, a homeland and a child are all seen as different degrees of the same monolithic quality of loss.

Kellehear (2005a, p 162) states:

> Those who know this kind of experience of bereavement [death of one's only child], who know this emptiness of heart that comes with deep loss, also *partly understand* the loss of country and identity that comes from the refugee, colonial or dementia experience, even if they are not literate about the relevant histories or biographies of those concerned. After all, loss is loss (emphasis added).

Or, death is death. The partial understanding of which Kellehear (2005a) speaks, that all people who know (deep) loss share a partial appreciation of all loss, is a vague idea because it is not clear what quality of loss is understood, what quality is only partially understood, and what quality is not understood at all. This universalistic view of loss not only flattens out the differences in degrees of loss and the circumstances of loss but also, in effect, hides the essential qualitative distinctions that these different degrees and circumstances express and entail. Universalising the quality of loss emphasises qualitative similarities at the expense of any qualitative distinctions that may obtain in any particular circumstance of loss. Universalising, by definition, is always an abstraction or decontextualisation in some measure.

Qualitative distinctions that are essential to the notion of loss can break up this monolithic construction of death and embrace critical subtleties in the meaning of death. These critical qualitative distinctions in death serve to emphasise not only death's contextual dependence but also, much more importantly, the nature of death itself and the quality to which death is opposed. Since death is opposed to birth, life or embodiment, qualitative distinctions in death obtain partly in order to understand, by contrast, the actual and symbolic meaning of birth, life or embodiment.

This is the explanation or justification for Kellehear (2005a) and palliative care to want to universalise loss, as a symbol of death as wise counsel, because the quality of loss has much to teach about materialistic acquisition or attachment to life, by qualitative contrast. Qualitative contrast allows language and symbolism some of its contextual and multidimensional richness, ambiguity and poetry. Identifying essential qualitative distinctions in death, therefore, is a key way to be able to comprehend and elucidate the full range of the meaning of death. And, consequently, this method of determining the essential qualitative distinctions in death is a key way to comprehend and elucidate the full range of the meaning of the birth–life–death cycle, circle or pathway.

The analysis discerns three essential qualitative distinctions in the idea of loss, and as a result, three qualitative distinctions in the idea of death. These three essential understandings are able to embrace the full range of the meaning of death and its contrasting quality, life, birth or embodiment. The primary task, therefore, is to discern and distinguish these three symbolic faces of death. The three interdependent and inseparable faces of death, the three necessary qualitative distinctions that death assumes, allow this expanded significance of death to be comprehended.

To conclude these introductory remarks, the three interdependent faces of death allow an inversion of romantically idealised conceptualisations of death. Romantic idealisations believe we need to correct our mistaken vision that sees only an illusory or provisionally negative side to death instead of the underlying, good and ever-present message of impermanence and the commonality of our human condition that death whispers. Our apparently mistaken vision interprets death's threat negatively when in reality death has our best interests at heart. This view argues that we see death wrongly when we perceive something sinister about death, since death is plainly 'normative and universal', although, as shown in Chapter Four, the meaning of normative is unclear in Kellehear (2005a, p 34). Being 'normative and universal', death must work for us not against us, despite appearances to the contrary. Romantic idealisations try to defang death, and so reduce it to a sentimental version of the age-old symbol of wise counsel that, as we shall see, involves a far more complex meaning than this sentimental version supposes.

SRV and the three faces of death

In SRV-based understanding, devaluation distinguishes between two types of inseparable and interdependent vulnerability. First, there is vulnerability from the risk of suffering *due to the (devalued) characteristic itself*, for example, from bodily suffering due to a physical disfigurement. Second, there is vulnerability from the risk of suffering *due to the harm done to the devalued person by others* (because of the devalued characteristic), for example, from suffering due to being mocked because of a physical disfigurement. In SRV theory, this second type of vulnerability is called the 'risk of devaluation'. Furthermore, the concept of devaluation is intersected by the SRV core theme of 'unconsciousness'. Because of this intersection, there are two types of devaluation, unconscious and conscious devaluation.

Wolfensberger (1992a) draws these interconnections and nuances together using a new term. Wolfensberger (1992a, p 1) coins the term 'deathmaking' from the French (*faire-mourir*) and German (*totmachen*) because there is no English word with the same discernment of nuance. While this fundamental and unifying concept of 'deathmaking' draws together the core of SRV theory, there is a greater significance in relation to understanding death. The concept of deathmaking connects ideas about death with SRV and ideas related to devaluation and the process of social stratification. The idea of deathmaking provides a formal means of understanding devaluation, and the vulnerability it involves, as having some sort of crucial connection with death.

Kellehear (2005a) defines loss in a romantic way, and consequently he defines death romantically to some degree. Loss is defined as the loss of something or someone cherished or possessed. By understanding death as the ultimate symbol of loss, anything and everything, any and every person, possessed or cherished holds the threat of loss and death. Loss of partner, child, pet, land, identity, ability, wealth, life, rationality, culture, home, love, innocence, freedom and so on – anything and everything implies loss by virtue of the mere embodiment or manifestation of the thing, and our possible attachment to it. Death is ever present in both the actual and symbolic sense. Loss then involves suffering. Deep loss involves "the emptiness of the heart" (Kellehear, 2005a, p 162).

However, this definition of loss tends to reduce the idea of loss to a universal of homogeneous quality. The idea of vulnerability, from or to loss, is able to expand this definition to allow the critical qualitative distinctions concerning loss to be seen. Only the limited notion of loss and death of Kellehear (2005a) and palliative care is able to be romantically idealised. As soon as loss is understood in the context of vulnerability to/from loss, a new quality of loss begins to appear.

Qualitative distinctions in loss

Besides the loss of something cherished, which loss can be romanticised, there is another altogether different quality to loss. The act of devaluation does not involve the loss of anything possessed. Although devaluation usually means the loss of many cherished things, these losses are the consequence of an overarching 'loss' characteristic of the act of devaluation. In the act of devaluation, our humanity is taken from us *by others*. The truth that we are human beings is denied, to varying degrees, because the act of devaluation presumes another person conceives of us as sub-human, less-than-human, other-than-human, used-to-be-human and so on. Devaluation is an extinction, a killing, a theft or a denial of that which cannot be 'lost'. Devaluation is a betrayal *by others* that aims to rob us of our humanity. Devaluation symbolically or actually kills us or, that is, 'makes us dead'. The losses due to devaluation are losses *imposed by others*.

There is nothing able to be idealised about this side to death. Romantic idealisation of any aspect of death necessarily devalues, denies or disregards this sinister side. Value or respect in the eyes of others is something bestowed *by others*, who acknowledge our equal or identical humanity, or denied *by others* who do not. And, since acts expressing devaluation deny, by definition, the absolute equality of our humanity at the level of values, devaluation is a killing, denial, betrayal or theft of one's humanity *by others*. Wolfensberger (1992a) uses the term 'deathmaking' to encode this insight in its essential, both actual and symbolic, correspondences with death. Seale (1998) also understands that symbolic killing is involved in acts of devaluation. Furthermore, he sees both actual and symbolic killing as "killing death", as a means to "sustain personal security about being in the world (ontological security)" (Seale, 1998, p 3). Seale's (1998) idea is perfectly clear yet paradoxical since it involves the idea of the 'death of death'. Such paradoxical meaning in death points to the need to refine qualitative distinctions in the idea of death to allow it to embrace these shades of meaning without recourse to paradox.

The act of devaluation can occur even without a person knowing it, for example, by someone inside a house laughing at a person with a disability as he/she passes by outside. The act of devaluation occurs to all of us to some degree because we all have some sort of characteristic that someone will want to devalue given half a chance. Every act of devaluation on any person with a similar devalued characteristic affects all devalued people in this group by reinforcing the social rectitude of the act. And devaluation of devalued people is unrelenting and inescapable. In these ways, the risk of devaluation causes an awareness of an ever-present vulnerability to arise. This is not a vulnerability to the 'loss' of humanity exactly, but to harm *by others*, to being made dead *by others*.

We cannot restore to ourselves that which is bestowed by others. One's humanity is not a cherished possession but the essential quality of being human. Alternatively, it is a cherished gift that is bestowed *by others* in deferential recognition of our identity in that humanity. The first two essential qualitative distinctions concerning loss are, therefore, the loss of something possessed and loss *imposed by others*.

Three faces of death

To review a little the logical development of this discussion so far, the new conceptualisation of vulnerability subsumes two qualitative distinctions in loss: vulnerability to a loss of something possessed or cherished and the vulnerability to the act of devaluation (and, therefore, to dehumanisation or harm *by others*). This latter vulnerability consists of a vulnerability to unconscious devaluation and a vulnerability to conscious devaluation. Just as Kellehear (2005a) associates a kind of 'compassion' with loss, there is also a greater compassion associated with this more refined conceptualisation of vulnerability. Since vulnerability subsumes loss, there is a compassion that subsumes the 'compassion' described by Kellehear (2005a). The discussion can only proceed once this confusion in terminology is clarified to take account of the necessary nuances in vulnerability.

Kellehear (2005a, p 88, p 93) connects his meaning of compassion with the sociological construct of 'solidarity' and with concepts like empathy. The connection with solidarity is more precise than the use of compassion. The following discussion uses the term 'solidarity' for Kellehear's term 'compassion', and reserves the use of 'compassion' for an all-embracing quality that includes solidarity, but also includes another facet of compassion that is essentially connected to the third qualitative distinction in loss. Before defining compassion in this sense, the third distinction in loss or vulnerability needs to be understood.

In order to explore this third distinction in loss, an unfashionable term, which is intrinsically involved in the idea of deathmaking, needs to be introduced. The step-wise building up of the nuances in vulnerability allows the meaning of this unfashionable term to appear.

Kellehear (2005a, p 85), citing Seale (1998) and Becker (1973), notes the sociological view that the vulnerability to death, "the organic susceptibility to death, is the main driving force behind all social and cultural activity". Such an analysis refers primarily to the first quality of vulnerability alone that reduces death to its physical manifestation. This materialistic view of death as the ultimate mediator of impermanence feeds directly into the idea of death as a modern deviance since death, as the immaterial, ever-present dark presence over one's shoulder, can have no meaning besides its connection with physical death or disembodiment. Death can, therefore, only be the terror to be assuaged, avoided or denied and, failing all else, romanticised as beneficial. The archetypal reaper's scythe lies in wait to dismember our bodies, in callous, even mischievous, disregard for the vulnerability of embodiment. Seeing death as deviant in the face of this apparently cold-hearted and merciless death is an understandable, although counterproductive, response that all of us have to address because of the vulnerability of our mere embodiment. Beginning from this abstract and materialistic version of the first face of death, death as the 'organic susceptibility of embodiment' alone, SRV-based understandings allow the nuances in vulnerability to be built up in three steps.

First, SRV theory understands that a certain vulnerability and suffering may, and often does, result from the devalued characteristic itself. For example, the suffering of lost capability from disability or dying is a direct suffering, arising from the disability or dying itself. That is, 'organic susceptibility of embodiment' is, or may be, itself a direct cause of suffering. This aspect might be termed *the vulnerability of embodiment*.

Second, SRV theory also understands that devaluation is a source of vulnerability to suffering at the hands of others and that there is an inseparable interdependence between the two vulnerabilities. This imposed vulnerability of our humanity is not the 'organic susceptibility of embodiment' itself. It is a higher order of suffering embedded *by others* into the 'vulnerability of embodiment'. This aspect might be termed *the vulnerability of human embodiment*.

Third, SRV theory via deathmaking takes this 'vulnerability of human embodiment' to the next and ultimate level. Deathmaking specifically differentiates between unintentional harm and intentional harm drawing both together under the banner of death. A term is required to differentiate between the unintentional and intentional types of deathmaking. The unfashionable term 'evil' includes all intentional harm to another, although certainly there is a qualified evil involved in unintentional harm. A lesser evil is a harm caused to another without the intent to harm, kill or make dead, without the necessary *mens rea* (literally, guilty mind). Unintentional harm is also evil, by virtue of the neglect of due concern to do no harm, or by virtue of the ignorance that harm is being done, and by virtue of the blamelessness of the victim. Although evil is an unfashionable term, it never goes out of style in devaluation and prejudice, particularly in politics and religion. Nevertheless, evil is a necessary category.

The ultimate deviance is not death, as the 'vulnerability of embodiment' or, that is, death as natural suffering and ultimate symbol of impermanence. Nor is death as the unintentional violation of the 'vulnerability of human embodiment' the ultimate deviance. Death as an instrument of evil, as intentional deathmaking, is the ultimate deviance. The third face of death is the face of evil. There is in evil the sense of a deliberate, self-satisfied attempt to violate the good in all people, or even to violate the goodness of existence itself. This aspect might be termed *the vulnerability of the principle of human embodiment*. Because of this evil in death, there is a certain symbolic necessity to somehow designate death as a deviance, which as we shall see, means there is also a certain symbolic necessity to somehow idealise death.

These three interdependent meanings of vulnerability are now able to be brought together under the aegis of death, in reverse order proceeding from the third face. Deathmaking subsumes all intentional harm, all evil. *The third face of death is intentional deathmaking.*

Deathmaking also subsumes all unintentional harm. *The second face of death is a fusion of both actual and symbolic deathmaking.*

And deathmaking subsumes all death that is not caused from either intentional or unintentional harm by others, because death 'is made' whenever death as impermanence occurs, either actually or symbolically. *The first face of death is virtual deathmaking.*

While Wolfensberger (1992a, pp 13-17) distinguishes six levels of "[d]irectness of [d]eathmaking" that add texture to the second face of death especially, he does not refer to virtual deathmaking. Death as impermanence is 'made' or imposed by no one. Being without intent, it operates as a virtual deathmaking. Actual or symbolic death due to impermanence is, in effect, a simulation, a virtuality, an illusion of deathmaking. This first face of death bears no malice, harbours no ill will. The first face of death does not intend to make us dead. Actually making us dead, or symbolically doing so through losses not imposed by others, is merely death's way of operating at this level, due to the impermanence of embodiment or manifestation. There is nothing evil about the first face of death.

By this means, by virtue of the innocence of its first face, death distinguishes itself from evil. Death becomes symbolically counterposed to evil, its third face, so that the final loss, the last step of existence, may be understood as free from any evil or beyond evil, in an ultimate way. The first face of death encodes the symbolic understanding that existence itself, the impermanence of existence itself, is free from evil. Moreover, since this face of death makes no exceptions, should all else fail to change a person who would do evil, the first face of death will non-discriminatorily and without malice obliterate this potential for evil. In this sense, the first face of death contains an ultimate symbol of the victory over evil, or the assurance of the defeat of evil. For this reason, it is not only natural but a symbolic necessity to idealise the first face of death. As a counterpoint to the evil third face of death, this first face of death is innocent, that is, non-discriminatory between good and evil (people and circumstances).

Seale's (1998, p 3) reference to the idea of "killing death" in the act of killing a person, whether actually or symbolically, gives a clear insight into the relative importance of death as impermanence compared to death as evil. That evil *can* in some critical way kill even death signifies that there is something in the evil intent of killing that seems able to transcend, defeat or deny death. Discussing Freud, Seale (1998, p 58) refers to killing others as "confirmation that one is indeed immune to death". In other words, the 'killing death' idea implies that there is a pseudo-immortality in evil, or killing others, that is somehow beyond death as the impermanence of embodiment. The idea of 'killing death' understands intent as the force that appears to allow some possibility of transcending death.

These symbolic meanings in the first face of death move directly into the playful, even innocent, imagery of the macabre and its dark romance and sense of humour. A skeleton dancing in macabre merriment on the grave is an ideal symbolic representation of the first face of death. Innocent playfulness works in partnership with what is most sublime in humanity. Halloween, 'All Hallows Eve', more in its Catholic than pagan meaning, encodes some important symbolic allusions in the first face of death. The living and the souls of the dead take on ghastly forms to scare away evil spirits. Halloween inaugurates the celebration of the saints, in All Saints' (Hallows) Day. By connecting in complex ways death, evil and sanctity, Halloween celebrates various facets of the victory over evil. The pseudo-immortality of evil in the third face of death becomes, thereby, counterposed to the immortality of sanctity. In this manner, the simple and direct fact of death as the impermanence of embodiment resonates with the other faces of death as keys to expanding the symbolic meaning of death.

From this brief excursion into the first face of death, a pattern can be discerned regarding the symbolism of death and its allusions can begin to be appreciated. The first face of death is innocent and 'good', ultimately or symbolically, with the connotation of being beyond good and evil in a non-discriminatory way. The second face of death is both good and evil, fused inseparably in and as existence. There is no clearer example of this fusion of good and evil than unintentional harm since its qualified evil derives from either a neutral or a good intention towards another. The third face of death is wanton evil, the disturbing face of self-satisfied evil. Since the three faces are interdependent and inseparable, we try to romanticise, exclude or deny any one part of this profound symbolism at the expense of death. Death, in its sublime sense, does not symbolise impermanence, suffering or loss. Death's essential meaning concerns its symbolic signification as the victory over evil, in its individual, social and universal senses. The connection of death with sanctity and the protective mantle of the saints through Halloween supports this contention.

Since the first face of death must be idealised to retain its symbolic implications, this discussion does not seek to dismiss palliative care's or Kellehear's (2005a) romantic idealisation of death but rather seeks to explain and refine it, just as this discussion also seeks to explain and refine the understanding of the deviance of death as a principle. Murder, the clearest example of intentional deathmaking, can serve to reiterate the central distinction regarding death as impermanence and evil. If a person is murdered, it is not death that kills but an evil, murderous intent. The first face of death does not kill in the same way that human beings do. The wound that is wilful murder injures the heart in far more harmful and complex ways than dying itself, due to the vulnerability of embodiment. A single murderous act can wreak havoc across the generations, whereas death as the impermanence of embodiment can leave a precious wound on the heart. This wound of love gives emotional force to romantic idealisation of death. Society's just responses to murderous acts also demonstrates the cruel harm done to the heart when human beings arrogate to themselves the power of death, which is, in some sense, a necessary feature of the human condition and human society.

Three faces of death and social processes

Wolfensberger (1992a, p 4) explains that an essential characteristic of all societies is social stratification since there has never been a society without stratification. Devaluation, as unconscious deathmaking, is an operative necessity of stratification since it is the obverse side of social valuation. The faces of death can, therefore, be related back to social processes.

The first quality of vulnerability is the vulnerability arising from the devalued characteristic itself. To repeat, this is death as impermanence or 'plain' suffering, ultimately and symbolically. The second quality of vulnerability is the vulnerability arising from unconscious devaluation. This is death as a fundamental and universal social process, both actually and symbolically. This is death as dehumanisation, or ultimately as symbolic non-existence. The third quality of vulnerability is the vulnerability arising from intentional devaluation. This is death as evil, murder ultimately, the symbol of 'actual non-existence'. This connection between evil and 'actual non-existence' indicates that evil is impossible, in some paradoxical or unique sense, because 'actual non-existence' cannot in any way exist, by definition.

Placing intentionality at the centre of the meaning of death, in the third face, inverts romantically idealised approaches that seek to place a materialistic abstraction of the first face of death at the centre. With intention as the central explanatory category able to embrace all nuances in the meaning of death, the third face of death becomes its foremost ever-present face, warning us not of impermanence but of the dangers in our potentiality to harm others, consciously and unconsciously. The wise counsel of the first face of death, which might advise us to help others, is altogether less urgent than that associated with the third face of death, which might advise us to stop injuring others. Failing to heed the counsel of the first face means we may neglect to do some good or continue to neglect our own best interests, whereas ignoring the counsel of the third face means that we may continue to directly do harm to others.

The second face of death intermingles with our every action since every act is either conscious/intentional or unconscious/unintentional and since every act can affect others towards valuing or devaluing them. A complex double meaning is entailed in the second face of death. The negative aspect, social devaluation, is opposed to the positive aspect, social valuation. Both processes are potentially relevant to every social interaction since social stratification is a fundamental fact of society. However, in the preceding derivation from vulnerability, only the negative aspect comes to describe the second face of death. The explanation is that death as a fundamental social process, as dehumanisation, is a direct and active instance of deathmaking. In other words, dehumanisation is readily seen as involving death somehow. Death as social valuation, on the other hand, appears to not be deathmaking, to simply involve the affirmation of life and to have nothing to do with death. However, every act of dehumanisation aims, in effect, to affirm the social value of the devaluing person or of some group valued by this person. Dehumanisation steals something of another's humanity in order to glorify one's own and try to transcend death. And every act of social valuation entails the potential for social devaluation. The unconsciousness of harm done by the positive, valuation side of this face of death means it cannot recognise its deathmaking impact. Only the negative aspect can reflect the complete symbolic meaning of this face of death since it can perceive all the deathmaking that is done. Because the negative, devaluation perspective is the victim's perspective, it perceives directly the harm done and allows the possibility to discern the intentionality or unintentionality of that harm. However, the valuation aspect, by virtue of its unconsciousness of devaluation can, at best, only reflect a partial understanding of the meaning of the second face of death, more like a self-made image of the second face of death seen through rose-coloured glasses.

Nonetheless, symbolic allusions in the valuation aspect of the second face of death remain powerful. Connecting living, humanisation and existence with unconsciousness regarding devaluation alludes to living, humanisation and existence as a mistaken, illusory and incomplete perspective. Living is dream-like, sleep-like or like being dead to the world. Since the devaluation aspect can comprehend the undistorted view of this face, symbolic non-existence and suffering *at the hands of others* are connected with the dispelling of unconsciousness or ignorance. Shortly, an example discussing 'identity politics', where specific groups "wish to make a virtue of one social difference" (Kellehear, 2005a, p 111), illustrates how the view from the valuation aspect can see only its own self-image in devalued people rather than being able to see from the devaluation perspective.

The idea of deathmaking inverts the materialistic way death is mostly conceptualised in late modernity and shows how the ultimate existential categories of good and evil subsume universalising ideas about death, life, suffering and loss. Recognition of the idea of deathmaking as an essential facet of death indicates the extent of the cost of romanticising death. Romanticised death, robbed of evil, cannot serve to symbolise the transformative victory over evil. The three faces of death have clear connections with several traditional religious explanations of human nature, reality and the purpose of society. As has been indicated, the view that the "organic susceptibility to embodiment" is "the main force driving all social and cultural processes" (Seale, 1998 and Becker, 1973, cited in Kellehear, 2005a, p 85) refers to the first face of death abstracted from its other two faces. However, the present analysis suggests this abstraction is an immense reduction of the idea of death, lacking the multidimensionality, ambiguity and immediacy that is unique to death. This discussion suggests that a far more complex triune face of death is the main force driving all social and cultural activity. By arrogating the power of death to ourselves, human beings actually and symbolically embody death to others, the ever-present threat of death at the hands of others being mediated by the processes of social stratification. This personification of death in the human being allows an ultimate vulnerability in each other's hands to be situated at the centre of what it means to be human. Under romantic idealisations, people can only personify death as the loss of someone/something cherished rather than personifying the radical and ambiguous otherness of death and evil that people also embody.

SRV considers the imperfectability of human beings and collectivities as the cause of social devaluation. SRV does not hypothesise further about why devaluation occurs or why power is exercised. Wolfensberger (1992a, p 3) has, however, explicitly identified the battle between good and evil in his conceptualisation of the human being – "the noble in them [human beings] pulls one way, the ignoble the other. So commonly, the flesh and the spirit are at war with each other". In contrast to social justice models or rights-based approaches to difference, SRV theory deliberately does not attribute the blame for devaluation to dominant groups of any description. SRV theory simply contends that we all devalue others and, to some degree, cannot avoid doing so. In addition, since no one can avoid being at risk of devaluation by others, vulnerability to devaluation is a universal experience.

At last, the three faces of death can be used to define compassion. Except in so far as romantic idealisations obscurely encode traditional religious meanings, they deny death its symbolic correspondence with the triumph over evil. Death works with and through human beings to make manifest sanctity and its antecedents. In this way, the triune face of death comes to refer to the highest purposes of human life. This is particularly pertinent to palliative care and its Christian ethos. Christ's resurrection of the body or embodiment, the victory over the universal first face of death, connects with His redemption of evil through His sacrificial death *at the hands of others*, in the third face of death. If evil, and the qualified evil that does not know what it is doing, is excluded from the conceptualisation of death by romanticising it, then sacrifice unto death in order to redeem evil can make no sense. Evil and death become disjoined, and the triumph over death as the enemy or adversary is reduced to an abstract acceptance of impermanence.

Just as one's humanity is a gift bestowed by others, intentional harm can only be removed or restored intentionally, that is, by an intentional good. This exceptional activity, the absolute end to the problem of evil is known as compassion or forgiveness. The harm one does to another can only be redeemed by forgiveness. This fundamentally religious concept understands that intentional harm is not just defeated by intentional self-sacrifice but redeemed. From the vantage point of forgiveness, evil is not simply without justification but without substance, as alluded to earlier when discussing the connection between evil and 'actual non-existence'.

Although this book asserts that death is devalued, there is one solitary exception where death is not only socially approved but glorified. Self-sacrificial deaths for the benefit of others are socially valued especially when redressing evil. The clearest example is death in war. Other examples include martyrdom and death while fighting crime or injustice. That such deaths remain socially valued in late modernity shows the essentiality of evil and the triumph over evil to the notion of death, and emphasises the exceptional nature of self-sacrificial dying for others.

All communities can only be founded on social justice. At the practical level, the necessity and absolute priority for justice to address harm done to people is a precondition for compassion to be meaningful. For devalued groups, since the risk of devaluation is relentless and inescapable, processes intended to be 'compassionate' can only be tainted by this embedded devaluation, as Chapter Four indicated. To give developing solidarity or empathy equal priority to redressing harm is to deny justice its prerogatives and proper domain, and also to deny compassion its just and proper meaning at the practical level. 'Compassionate' communities, founded on empathy or solidarity, are romantic idealisations or utopian abstractions, as Kellehear (2005a) recognises. Compassion is primarily an inner act, the inner redemptive or unitive act. It is an intentional choice to forgive evil or harm done to one. In a sense it is to take this suffering or evil upon oneself. A society that prioritises turning the other cheek ahead of justice in any way is an abstraction because, were any society able to be founded on self-sacrifice in the face of evil, then that society is not going to be around for long. Besides, all societies have a responsibility to protect their members and uphold the rights of innocent victims of crime, since this act of justice is the proper expression of compassion at the practical level. Seeking to develop an empathic understanding of the commonality of loss views loss as if it were a mere fact of life that did not also involve a risk to harm by others. A shared sense of loss imposed by others has many times been the cause not of compassion but of wars of revenge. In contrast, the first principles of SRV understand that we are all actual and potential perpetrators of devaluation and all actual and potential victims of devaluation. In other words, SRV theory explains that while loss due to a fact of life, such as some disabilities or some deaths, may be a cause of suffering, the greater suffering is that we impose additional losses onto people experiencing such facts of life as a fundamental feature of the nature of society and the individual.

To the extent that both palliative care and public health approaches are not grounded in the explicit commitment to address devaluation before all else, these approaches attempt to put the cart before the horse. As has been shown, both palliative care and public health approaches to end-of-life care provide clear evidence of the unconsciousness of devaluation embedded into them. Both in principle and in practice, only the negative devaluation perspective, in the second face of death, can embrace the whole picture. Unless SRV theory is used to reveal devaluation, positive valuation perspectives that seek to embed positive ideals into existing social processes must almost certainly increase the devaluation in these processes. Furthermore, as shown in Chapter Four, such artificially embedded processes disguise this devaluation as goodness, thereby perpetuating devaluation while intending to do the opposite. The valuation perspective can, and often does, unconsciously believe its own publicity. While the devaluation perspective has the possibility of seeing the harm done, and the intentionality or unintentionality of that harm, the positive valuation perspective has no possibility of seeing the harm, unless it involves intentional harm.

The positive valuation perspective cannot see its own unconsciousness, by definition. This perspective has no possibility of seeing anything other than its own illusory constructs or self-image. There is another critical prerogative of the devaluation perspective in the second face of death concerning this unconsciousness. Eventually, the devaluation perspective has the possibility and right to draw a line in the sand where it chooses to disbelieve the unintentionality of devaluation and invoke the principle of jurisprudence that 'ignorance of the law is no excuse'. The devaluation perspective can invoke its right before the law and refuse to accept that unconscious devaluation is blame-free or unpunishable, simply because it is unintentional. This principle validates the right to resist devaluation and judge blameworthy those who are apparently ignorant of the harm being done. From the devaluation perspective, someone must eventually take the responsibility for relentless, inescapable devaluation.

The person who is unconsciously devaluing another can see nothing wrong in what he/she is doing. Nevertheless, his/her seemingly good acts are unjust acts from the devalued person's perspective, *which is that of the law*, because he/she abuses the devalued person's humanity, because this is the effect of devaluing acts irrespective of intent. The law takes the place of the devaluing person's conscience and seeks first to stop the harm, and then, by punishment, to try to force on him/her an awareness of the effects of what he/she is doing. In social processes, justice must precede compassion.

The devaluation perspective should take precedence over all other approaches and inform them, since only this perspective can be true, in the sense of being able to take into account both the devalued and valued person's perspective. No society has ever included 'all people'. A perspective addressed to 'all people' or to 'social inclusion' in communities as a whole is, in effect, an encryption of the dominant valuation perspective designed to perpetuate the devaluation of vulnerable people. In 1866 Howe states: "Nowhere is wisdom more necessary than in the guidance of charitable impulses. Meaning well is only half our duty; thinking right is the other and equally important half" (cited in Wolfensberger, 1975, p 19). Wisdom, as in Solomon's case, involves right discernment regarding intentionality toward vulnerable people.

The following example illustrates the illusory character of the valuation perspective in the second face of death. Kellehear's (2005a, pp 111–12) discussion of 'identity politics' appears to inform, at least in part, his view that an exclusive focus on abnormality or difference limits the reach, effectiveness and workability of normalisation or approaches that solely address devaluation. SRV theory distinguishes itself from and has its own significant problems with 'identity politics', as illustrated by Wolfensberger's (1999, 2002) discussion of rights-based approaches to disability. One such problem is that rights-based approaches misunderstand devaluation by focusing on power and blaming dominant groups. A second problem is that "having power is definitely not the same thing as being either valued, or even accepted, by others" (Wolfensberger, 2002, p 254). The following discussion, therefore, does not seek to defend the "conflict model" (Wolfensberger, 2002, p 253) of 'identity politics' but rather to explain a certain inevitability and prerogative of difference-based resistance by devalued people.

Kellehear (2005a, p 112) quotes Anthias and Yuval-Davis (1992, p 194): "establishing a system of identity politics as a form of resistance to Eurocentrism, Orientalism and racism fails exactly because its basic assumptions have been formed within a discourse of difference it wants to attack". Kellehear (2005a, p 112) explains that "hence, the threats to ... compassionate policies from identity politics then come from singular rather than dual strategies of resistance". He means that, if applied on its own, the strategy of "challenging their [dominant groups'] aversion to difference" threatens compassion by pointing the finger and emphasising differences. However, if combined with "demonstrating the universal traits and experiential connections we have in common with each other" (Kellehear, 2005a, p 112), the dual strategy can obviate the threat.

This view implies three inappropriate assumptions. First, it implies that devalued people do not understand that resistance based on challenging the aversion to difference of dominant groups is counterproductive, when devalued people's lives constantly prove both the futility and increasing danger of such resistance. The mere existence of devalued people is evidence to the devaluing mentality that devalued people are challenging dominant groups' aversion to difference. Alternatively, this view implies devalued people do not know they are colluding with a 'discourse of difference'. Since every action or inaction by a devalued person proves his/her difference to the devaluing mentality (Elliot, 1996), a devalued person's mere existence necessarily colludes with this discourse, and there is, therefore, no clearer fact to a devalued person.

Second, this view implies that the flawed difference-based strategy of devalued people plays some sort of role in exacerbating devaluation or failing to defeat it. Using the example of racism, this view appears to blame, in part, the continuance of racism, or the failure to defeat it, on the victims of racism. In other words, if devalued people would act, feel or think differently then they would not be so devalued (by racism), or they could work more effectively against devaluation (racism) and defeat it. The irrationality and unconsciousness of racism, not to mention its evil, denies, by definition, any rational or discursive attempt to counter it. Adopting a discourse that tries to engage or step around this irrationality, unconsciousness and evil in order to focus on commonalities must collude with it in a far more dangerous and insidious manner than directly challenging it within its own discourse.

Third, this view implies that efforts to emphasise commonalities are not made or are made counterproductively within a discourse of difference. Irrespective of the discourse devalued people adopt, they are forced to try in every way imaginable to embody the commonalities valued by the dominant group's mindset. The more devalued people threaten to succeed and exhibit shared commonalities, the more their 'advancement' is resented as the very worst kind of difference because devalued people are trying to arrogate to themselves that which can only belong to the dominant group. Since devalued people live this dead-end reality every day, they know that they can do nothing to escape this vicious circle. Inevitably and finally, devalued people have no choice but to challenge evil as evil and unconscious 'evil' as injustice.

The central flaw, therefore, in the argument that directly resisting a 'discourse of difference' embodies, supports or engages its assumptions is that it presumes there is some other discourse that devalued people might adopt. Oppression consists in the exclusion or violent eradication of all discourse other than that of difference. Devalued people have no choice, cannot help but resist, as Wolfensberger (1992a, p 12) notes. By their mere existence or finally by some deliberate means, devalued people inevitably resist devaluation. Much so-called challenging, settling-in or disturbing behaviour in institutional care is individual and group resistance to the oppression intrinsic to segregated environments.

Jane Elliot's (1996) discrimination workshops have to publicly dehumanise oppressors, who have been artificially placed in the role of oppressed people, in order that they can come to understand in some small way that there is no action or inaction by a devalued person that does not confirm a 'discourse of difference'. The oppressed person can win an inner victory in his/her own mind and, indeed, must do so if he/she is to get through each second. However, although the devalued person can win an inner victory, oppressors will not know, much less care, and certainly will not change one iota as a result (Elliot, 1996). SRV would add that only the 'subliminally' persuasive effects from enhancing image and competency can have any impact until a devalued person occupies a valued role. Only from that point can his/her plain actions have any chance of being able to not confirm his/her difference, although it is still the 'subliminally' persuasive impact on mindsets of positive expectancies associated with the valued role itself that has the critical effect rather than any coercive means.

Unless plainly or purely evil, which seems a virtual impossibility since almost all evil appears to imagine that some good of some sort is being served, the devaluing mindset is either unconscious of its devaluation, or it mistakes evil for good. For example, in ethnic cleansing, mass slaughter is believed a virtuous act to protect one's own ethnic group. In both cases, this mindset sees nothing wrong, so there is no possibility of it wanting to be different, especially, in the first case, with the incentives of valued group membership and, in the second case, with the additional incentive of the salacious pleasure from harming others and wielding the power of death.

The problem with emphasising human commonalities is that a shared commonality, if realised, simply becomes another cause of division and another reason to devalue some other person or group.

> Individuals are very much at odds with each other. And when individuals form collectivities on the basis of some bond or some characteristic that they share, the very thing that draws the members of such a collectivity together almost automatically becomes the bone of contention that divides them from other persons who are not members, and especially from other collectivities. (Wolfensberger, 1992a, p 3)

This discussion has barely scratched the surface of the triune face of death and its implications. Death has a unique and most potent symbolic power, especially through its connections with redemption and the victory over evil. Death is the ultimate symbol of paradox and ambiguity. Death as time exists in an evanescent present, which dies as it is born. Christian redemption suggests that Christ's death defeats death. The triune face of death provides a key to unlock the profound symbolic meaning of death. From the perspective of triune death, death is not a mere fact of existence nor a merciless destruction of embodiment but a quality of existence that places intention and vulnerability to harm by others at the centre of the drama of human life. Death is not so much a punishment as a gift, and not so much a gift as a victory, consciously wrought in the human heart.

EIGHT

The choice

SRV crossover into palliative care

This book aims to provide the theoretical groundwork to enable the palliative care field to begin to analyse the current conceptualisation of palliative care from an entirely new perspective.

SRV's crossover into palliative care enables the palliative care system to become aware of its perpetuation of the devaluation of people who are dying and how to address this devaluation. To this point, explorations in end-of-life care by SRV proponents have focused on protecting vulnerable people's lives rather than on palliative care specifically. Some projects of the interdisciplinary research work of the New Emerging Teams Research Project (Canadian Institutes of Health Research, 2003) represent, to the author's knowledge, the first significantly funded research project with crossover between SRV and palliative care. As part of this project, Lutfiyya (2003) aims to develop "a conceptual analysis of how social devaluation and SRV fit into palliative and end-of-life care". Unpublished work by van Bommel (2003) has involved the assessment of some palliative care services using SRV-based criteria. To the author's knowledge, his own work, together with van Bommel's around the same time in the mid- to late 1990s, represents the first SRV-based evaluations of specific palliative care services. This book hopes to further this crossover by formally bringing SRV theory to bear on the current conceptualisation of palliative care. Kellehear's (2005a, pp 30-5) introduction of a critique of normalisation theory, and some aspects of SRV, regarding end-of-life care is a further recent development.

Two future paths

Palliative care faces a choice similar to the one faced in the intellectual disability services system 30-40 years ago. Unless palliative care radically alters its social organisation and practice, it can only continue to unconsciously harm people who are dying by devaluing them.

The proof of the functionality of deinstitutionalised systems by the intellectual disability services system becomes even more persuasive when the outcomes necessary for a deinstitutionalised palliative care system are understood to be far simpler than those required in the intellectual disability sector. Unlike people with an intellectual disability, people who are dying, for the most part, are established in valued roles and have valued histories. The key need is simply to defend the valued role of living at home against the threat of institutionalisation.

At bottom, there can only be one explanation for the system's failure to fulfil the wish of the overwhelming majority to die at home. The health, aged and palliative care systems are constructed in such a way as to deny this wish, otherwise a different outcome would result. Only the most socially valued can step outside this system with its inexorable pull toward an institutional death, and ensure the wish to die at home is fulfilled. The impact of the health, aged and palliative care systems on dying at home is brought into question when, with reference to Australia for example, it is estimated that "less than 1 per cent of people over the age of 65 years die by choice in their own homes" (Stevens et al, 2000, p 180).

Saunders' marriage of religion and medicine in one institution for people who are dying makes a very loud and authoritative statement that the modern deviance of dying is under total control. However, this book repeatedly stresses that an institutional model applies not only to an institution itself but also applies to the philosophy and its institutional programme of care on which the institution is founded. For example, approaches that concentrate service provision in one agency, or provide services across many aspects of life, or collect devalued people together for programmes, or simulate valued living patterns, or separate people from their valued community, or duplicate available generic services, are institutional whether they occur in an institution, a private home or anywhere else. All these institutional approaches are generally applied by community-based palliative care services and are not just the province of hospices, nursing homes or inpatient palliative care units.

Saunders aims to develop a hospice as something between a private home and a hospital (Saunders, 1977). The aim of hospice houses is the same. A home can be turned into an institution virtually completely in terms of the services provided therein. However, an institution can be made like a home in only relatively tokenistic ways that are necessarily counterfeit simulations of valued ways of living at home. No matter how home-like we try to make a hospice (or hospice house), it will always and essentially be an institution. However, the home can fully remain a home while incorporating hospital-like or hospice-like services, provided institutional approaches are not imposed on it.

In comparing a home to an institution as a site of care, the essential qualitative difference between them is that an institution of care is a specially created setting for devalued people only. Because the institution of care is a specially created residential facility and not a private home, a person must be institutionalised in order to live in an institution. This act, by definition, necessitates the loss of home and community and the pre-existing valued social roles occupied or signified therein. The assumptions, contents and processes of institutions, such as hospices and inpatient units, are not just different in degree to those in the organisational form called the private home, they are of an entirely different kind.

Without institutions for ageing, disability, chronic conditions or dying, the future landscape of care looks very different from what we see today. The future of chronic care and related systems lies in making the home the centre of care. In that future, people in their homes are directly funded to access the supports they choose in order to live valued lives. A range of generic home support services provides various sorts of direct assistance to a wide variety of groups. These services adopt a 'whatever-it-takes' approach to enabling or maintaining valued lives and work in cooperation with existing professional community resources such as primary, community and public health services and local physiotherapy, complementary therapy and religious organisations.

Other community elements such as local retailers, trades people, service organisations, educational bodies, recreational groups, churches and governments also offer a variety of support opportunities for people. Neighbourhoods and communities develop novel and highly responsive support patterns for people needing assistance, when these innovations are guided by SRV principles and the experience of people at high risk of devaluation, such as people with HIV/AIDS. Generic home and community support facilitators work with people needing assistance, and their families/carers, to spend the funds directly provided to people in ways that support their dreams and personal circumstances. These facilitators work with friends, neighbours, communities, organisations and services to build an interconnected support network. Specialist services, such as palliative care services, work with such generic facilitators and people needing support, assisting with advocacy and monitoring quality of support, as well as ensuring accountability of the support received. Specialist services work with educational organisations to provide education for service providers, organisations and individuals in specialised areas such as palliative care. Users and concerned citizens form a variety of voluntary and paid generic advocacy bodies and organisations that assist in driving the provision of support toward highly responsive approaches. All approaches aim to copy the 'culturally valued analogue' for each particular context.

SRV theory should be used to direct the understanding and development of palliative and end-of-life care in order to redress the social devaluation of people who are dying or ageing. At the philosophical level, the triune face of death can serve as a guide for palliative care in examining its understanding of death and suffering. This new conceptualisation of death allows the clarification of many misconceptions around the meaning of death and allows the philosophical basis of end-of-life and palliative care to grapple with the paradoxes in the present romantic and universalistic conceptualisations of death.

Social and cultural processes are not driven by death as 'the vulnerability of embodiment' but by death as 'vulnerability as such', in all its facets. This vulnerability confronts us as the eternal tension between good and evil, symbolised by the interdependence of the three faces of death. Triune death offers a new way to understand modern dilemmas and contradictions in prevailing views about death and dying. The three faces of death locate devaluation, difference and evil as the central domain of death and the critical perspective to be understood.

References

Addams, S. (1993) 'A gendered history of the social management of death and dying in Foleshill, Coventry, during the inter-war years', in D. Clark (ed) *The sociology of death: Theory, culture and practice*, Oxford: Blackwell, pp 149-68.

Ahmedzai, S. (1993) 'The medicalisation of dying: A doctor's view', in D. Clark (ed) *The future for palliative care*, Buckingham: Open University Press, pp 140-7.

Alaszewski, A. and Wun, W. (1994) 'Residential services', in N. Malin (ed) *Implementing community care*, Buckingham: Open University Press, pp 157-73.

Anleu, S. (1995) *Deviance, conformity and control* (2nd edn), Melbourne: Longman.

Anthias, F. and Yuval-Davis, N. (1992) *Racialized boundaries*, London: Routledge.

Aranda, S. (1993) *What is the relationship between palliative care philosophy and care received by dying clients and their primary caregivers? A qualitative evaluation of the Melbourne Citymission Hospice*, Melbourne: Melbourne Citymission Hospice Service.

Arendt, H. (1963) *Eichmann in Jerusalem: A report on the banality of evil*, New York, NY: Vintage Press.

Argyris, C. (1985) *Strategy, change and defense routines*, Boston, MA: Pitman Publishing.

Aries, P. (1974) *Western attitudes toward death*, London: Marion Boyars.

Aries, P. (1981) *The hour of our death*, London: Allen Lane.

Backer, B., Hannon, N. and Russell, N. (1982) *Death and dying: Individuals and institutions*, New York, NY: John Wiley and Sons.

Baer, E. and Lowery, B. (1987) 'Patient and situational factors that affect nursing students' like or dislike of caring for patients', *Nursing Research*, vol 36, no 5, pp 298-302.

Baider, L. (1972) 'Some observations on the process of dying', *Australian Journal of Social Issues*, vol 7, no 3, pp 207-16.

Bailey, B. (1988) *Almshouses*, London: Robert Hale.

Baldwin, S. and Hattersley, J. (eds) (1991) *Mental handicap: Social science perspectives*, London: Tavistock/Routledge.

Baly, M. (1987) 'The Nightingale nurses: The myth and the reality', in C. Maggs (ed) *Nursing history: The state of the art*, London: Croom Helm, pp 33-59.

Bank-Mikkelson, N. (1980) 'Denmark', in R. Flynn and K. Nitsch (eds) *Normalization, social integration, and community services*, Baltimore, MD: University Park Press, pp 51-70.

Barr, O. (1993) 'Reap the benefits of a co-operative approach', *Professional Nurse*, vol 8, no 7, pp 473-77.

Baum, D. (1998) 'Introduction: The magnitude of the problem', in A. Goldman (ed) *Care of the dying child*, Oxford: Oxford University Press, pp 1-13.

Bayley, M. (1991) 'Normalisation or social role valorization: An adequate philosophy?', in S. Baldwin and J. Hattersley (eds) *Mental handicap: Social science perspectives*, London: Tavistock/Routledge, pp 87-99.

Becker, E. (1973) *The denial of death*, New York, NY: Free Press.

Biswas, B. (1993) 'The medicalization of dying: a nurse's view', in D. Clark (ed) *The future for palliative care*, Buckingham: Open University Press, pp 132-9.

Blouin, A., Lewis, J., Malone, N. and Metz, K. (1996) 'Improving quality through nursing case management', in D. Flarey and S. Blancett (eds) *Handbook of nursing case management: Health care delivery in a world of managed care*, Gaithersburg, MD: Aspen Publishers, pp 170-83.

Bosanquet, N. and Salisbury, C. (eds) (1999) *Providing a palliative care service: Towards an evidence base*, Oxford: Oxford University Press.

Boschma, G. (1997) 'Ambivalence about nursing's expertise: the role of a gendered holistic ideology in nursing 1890-1990', in A. Rafferty, J. Robinson and R. Elkan (eds) *Nursing history and the politics of welfare*, London: Routledge, pp 164-76.

Bowling, A. (1983) 'The hospitalisation of death: Should more people die at home?', *Journal of Medical Ethics*, vol 9, no 3, pp 158-61.

Bradshaw, A. (1996) 'The spiritual dimension of hospice: The secularization of an ideal', *Social Science and Medicine*, vol 43, no 3, pp 409-19.

Bray, J. (1996) 'A-Z of creative therapies', in R. Fisher and P. McDaid (eds) *Palliative day care*, London: Arnold, pp 198-221.

Brown, H. and Smith, H. (eds) (1992) *Normalisation: A reader for the nineties*, London: Tavistock/Routledge.

Buber, M. (1961) *Between man and man*, translated and introduced by Ronald Gregor Smith, London: Collins.

Buber, M. (1970) *I and thou: A new translation with a prologue 'I and you' and notes by Walter Kaufmann*, New York, NY: Scribner.

Canadian Institutes of Health Research (2003) 'Palliative and end of life care: New emerging team grants', accessed 2 July 2006 (www.cihr-irsc.gc.ca/e/15921.html, www.hsf.ca/research/competition/FundInitiatives/Palliative.html).

Card, L. (1999) 'The shift to family and community: The story of Xavier's Children's Support Network', in A. Cross, J. Sherwin, P. Collins, B. Funnell and M. Rodgers (eds) *Gathering the wisdom: Changing realities in the lives of people with disabilities*, Brisbane: CRU Publications, pp 50-61.

Carey, D. (1986) *Hospice inpatient environments: Compendium and guidelines*, New York, NY: Van Nostrand Reinhold Company.

Carlin, M. (1989) 'Medieval English hospitals', in L. Granshaw and R. Porter (eds) *The hospital in history*, London: Routledge, pp 21-40.

Carpenter, M. (1980) 'Asylum nursing before 1914: A chapter in the history of labour', in C. Davies (ed) *Rewriting nursing history*, London: Croom Helm, pp 123-46.

Cartwright, A. (1993) 'Dying when you're old', *Age and Ageing*, vol 22, no 6, pp 425-30.

Cartwright, F. (1977) *A social history of medicine*, London: Longman.

Carveth, J. (1995) 'Perceived patient deviance and avoidance by nurses', *Nursing Research*, vol 44, no 3, pp 173-78.

Charmaz, K. (1980) *The social reality of death: Death in contemporary America*, Reading, MA: Addison-Wesley Publishing Company.

Church, O. (1987) 'The emergence of training programs for asylum nursing at the turn of the century', in C. Maggs (ed) *Nursing history: The state of the art*, London: Croom Helm, pp 107-23.

Clark, D. (1993) 'Whither the hospices?', in D. Clark (ed) *The future for palliative care*, Buckingham: Open University Press, pp 167-77.

Clark, D. (nd) 'Hospice in historical perspective', *Encyclopedia of Death and Dying*, accessed 10 July 2006 (www.deathreference.com/Ho-Ka/Hospice-in-Historical-Perspective.html).

Clark, D. and Seymour, J. (1999) *Reflections on palliative care*, Buckingham: Open University Press.

Clark, K. (1996) 'Alternate case management models', in D. Flarey and S. Blancett (eds) *Handbook of nursing case management: Health care delivery in a world of managed care*, Gaithersburg: Aspen Publishers, pp 295-304.

Cohen, S., Mount, B., Tomas, J. and Mount, L. (1996) 'Existential well-being is an important determinant of quality of life: Evidence from the McGill Quality of Life Questionnaire', *Cancer*, vol 77, no 3, pp 576-86.

Connor, S. (1998) *Hospice: Practice, pitfalls and promise*, Washington, DC: Taylor & Francis.

Conrad, P. and Schneider, J. (1980) *Deviance and medicalization: From badness to sickness*, St Louis, MO: Mosby.

Corley, M. and Goren, S. (1998) 'The dark side of nursing: Impact of stigmatising responses on patients', *Scholarly Inquiry for Nursing Practice*, vol 12, no 2, pp 99-122.

Corner, J. and Dunlop, R. (1997) 'New approaches to care', in D. Clark, J. Hockley and S. Ahmedzai (eds) *New themes in palliative care*, Buckingham: Open University Press, pp 288-302.

Covenant Hospice (2007) Pensacola, accessed 31 January (www.covenanthospice.org/).

Cowles, E. (1887) 'Nursing reform for the insane', *American Journal of Insanity*, vol 44, no 2, pp 176-91.

Crichton, A. (1990) *Slowly taking control? Australian governments and healthcare provision, 1788-1988*, Sydney: Allen and Unwin.

Crowther, M. (1981) *The workhouse system 1834-1929: The history of an English social institution*, London: Batsford Academic and Educational.

Cummins, C. (1968) 'The administration of lunacy and idiocy in New South Wales, 1788-1855', *Australian Studies in Health Service Administration, No 2*, Monograph, Sydney: University of New South Wales.

Deegan, P. (1990) 'Spirit breaking: When the helping professions hurt', *The Humanistic Psychologist*, vol 18, no 3, pp 301-13.

de Swaan, A. (1990) *The management of normality: Critical essays in health and welfare*, London: Routledge.

DeVellis, B., Adams, J. and DeVellis, R. (1984) 'Effects of information on patient stereotyping', *Research in Nursing and Health*, vol 7, no 3, pp 237-44.

DiMaggio, P. and Powell, W. (1983) 'The iron cage revisited: Institutional isomorphism and collective rationality in organizational fields', *American Sociological Review*, vol 48, no 2, pp 147-60.

Doty, P. (2000) *Cost-effectiveness of home and community-based long-term services*, Washington, DC: US Department of Health and Human Services, Washington Office of Disability, Aging and Long-Term Care Policy, accessed 18 July 2003 (http://aspe.hhs.gov/daltcp/reports/costeff.htm).

Douglas, C. (1992) 'For all the saints', *British Medical Journal*, vol 304, no 6826, p 579.

Doyle, D. (1990) 'Facing the 1990s: special issues', *Hospice Update*, vol 2, no 1, pp 1-9.

Doyle, D. (1995) 'The future of palliative care', in I. Corless, B. Germino and M. Pittman (eds) *A challenge for living: Dying, death, and bereavement*, Boston, MA: Jones and Bartlett, pp 377-91.

Doyle, D. (1999) *Upon reflection: A farewell address delivered at Geneva, Switzerland 25 September 1999*, Houston, TX: International Association for Hospice and Palliative Care, accessed 18 July 2003 (http://hospicecare.com/DDFarewell.htm).

Duffy, D. (1995) 'Out of the shadows: A study of the special observation of suicidal psychiatric in-patients', *Journal of Advanced Nursing*, vol 21, no 5, pp 944-50.

Dumont, M. (1994) 'Genesis of a community psychiatrist', in W. Kornblum and C. Smith (eds) *The healing experience: Readings on the social context of health care*, Englewood Cliffs, NJ: Prentice Hall, pp 34-41.

Early, T. and Poertner, J. (1995) 'Examining current approaches to case management for families with children who have serious emotional disorders', in B. Friesen and J. Poertner (eds) *From case management to service coordination for children with emotional, behaviour and mental disorders: Building on family strengths*, Baltimore, MD: Paul H. Brookes Publishing, pp 37-62.

Elliot, J. (1996) 'Blue eyed', video recording, produced by C. Strigel and B. Verhaag, directed by B. Verhaag, Denkmal Filmproduction, Germany.

Ellis, J. and Luckasson, R. (1984) 'Hospice and the devaluation of human life: A response', *Mental Retardation*, vol 22, no 4, pp 163-4.

Evans, D. (1983) 'The plight of the poor in the working-man's paradise', in J. Pearn and C. O'Carrigan (eds) *Australia's quest for colonial health: Some influences on early health and medicine in Australia*, Brisbane: University of Queensland, pp 203-12.

Ferleger, D. and Boyd, P. (1980) 'Anti-institutionalization: The promise of the Pennhurst case', in R. Flynn and K. Nitsch (eds) *Normalization, social integration, and community services*, Baltimore, MD: University Park Press, pp 141-66.

Field, D. (1989) *Nursing the dying*, London: Tavistock/Routledge.

Field, D. and James, N. (1993) 'Where and how people die', in D. Clark (ed) *The future for palliative care*, Buckingham: Open University Press, pp 6-29.

Field, D. and Johnson, I. (1993) 'Volunteers in the British hospice movement', in D. Clark (ed) *The sociology of death: Theory, culture and practice*, Oxford: Blackwell, pp 198-217.

Field, D., Hockey, J. and Small, N. (1997) 'Making sense of difference: Death, gender and ethnicity in modern Britain', in D. Field, J. Hockey and N. Small (eds) *Death, gender and ethnicity*, London: Routledge, pp 1-28.

Fisher, R. (1991) 'Introduction: Palliative care – a rediscovery', in J. Penson and R. Fisher (eds) *Palliative care for people with cancer*, London: Edward Arnold, pp 3-9.

Fisher, R. (1996) 'Restorative gardens', in R. Fisher and P. McDaid (eds) *Palliative day care*, London: Edward Arnold, pp 83-4.

Flanagan, J. and Holmes, S. (1999) 'Facing the issue of dependence: Some implications from the literature for the hospice and hospice nurses', *Journal of Advanced Nursing*, vol 29, no 3, pp 592-9.

Flynn, R. and Lemay, R. (eds) (1999) *A quarter century of normalization and Social Role Valorization: Evolution and impact*, Ottawa: University of Ottawa Press.

Flynn, R. and Nitsch, K. (eds) (1980) *Normalization, social integration, and community services*, Baltimore, MD: University Park Press.

Foucault, M. (1973) (translated by A.M. Sheridan) *The birth of the clinic: An archaeology of medical perception*, London: Tavistock.

Foucault, M. (1988) (translated by R. Howard) *Madness and civilisation: A history of insanity in the age of reason*, New York, NY: Vintage Books.

Franks, P. (1999) 'Need for palliative care', in N. Bosanquet and C. Salisbury (eds) *Providing a palliative care service: Towards an evidence base*, Oxford: Oxford University Press, pp 43-56.

Freud, S. (1915) 'Thoughts for the times on war and death', reprinted (1953-1974) in the *Standard Edition of the Complete Psychological Works of Sigmund Freud* (trans. and ed. J. Strachey), vol 14, London: Hogarth Press.

Friere, P. (1972) *Cultural action for freedom*, Harmondsworth: Penguin.

Friesen, B. and Briggs, H. (1995) 'The organization and structure of service coordination mechanisms', in B. Friesen and J. Poertner (eds) *From case management to service coordination for children with emotional, behaviour and mental disorders: Building on family strengths*, Baltimore, MD: Paul H. Brookes Publishing, pp 63-94.

Froggatt, K. (1997) 'Order in disorder: Rites of passage in the hospice culture', *Mortality*, vol 2, no 2, pp 123-36.

Froggatt, K. and Walter, T. (1995) 'Hospice logos', *Journal of Palliative Care*, vol 11, no 4, pp 39-47.

Fulton, R. (1972) 'Death and dying: Some sociological aspects of terminal care', *Modern Medicine*, May 29, pp 74-7.

Gamlin, R. (1998) 'An exploration of the meaning of dignity in palliative care', *European Journal of Palliative Care*, vol 5, no 6, pp 187-90.

Gardner, J. and Glanville, L. (2005) 'New forms of institutionalization in the community', in K. Johnson and R. Traustadóttir (eds) *Deinstitutionalization and people with intellectual disabilities: In and out of institutions*, London: Jessica Kingsley Publishers, pp 220-30.

Germino, B. (1995) 'Dying at home', in I. Corless, B. Germino and M. Pittman (eds) *A challenge for living: Dying, death, and bereavement*, Boston, MA: Jones and Bartlett, pp 69-76.

Gibson, D. (1984a) 'Hospice and the new devaluation of human life', *Mental Retardation*, vol 22, no 4, pp 157-62.

Gibson, D. (1984b) 'Rejoinder', *Mental Retardation*, vol 22, no 4, p 169.

Glaser, B. and Strauss, A. (1965) *Awareness of dying*, London: Weidenfeld and Nicolson.

Glaser, B. and Strauss, A. (1968) *Time for dying*, Chicago, IL: Aldine.

Glickman, M. (1997) 'Making palliative care better: Quality improvement, multi-professional audit and standards', *Occasional Paper 12*, London: National Council for Hospice and Specialist Palliative Care Services.

Godden, J. (1997) '"For the benefit of mankind": Nightingale's legacy and hours of work in Australian nursing, 1868-1939', in A. Rafferty, J. Robinson and R. Elkan (eds) *Nursing history and the politics of welfare*, London: Routledge, pp 177-91.

Goldman, A. (ed) (1998) *Care of the dying child*, Oxford: Oxford University Press.

Gordon, A. (1984) 'Reaction to Gibson', *Mental Retardation*, vol 22, no 4, pp 164-6.

Gordon, A. (1996) 'Hospice and minorities: A national study of organizational access and practice', *The Hospice Journal*, vol 11, no 1, pp 49-69.

Gorer, G. (1965) *Death, grief and mourning in contemporary Britain*, London: Cresset Press.

Granshaw, L. (1989a) 'Introduction', in L. Granshaw and R. Porter (eds) *The hospital in history*, London: Routledge, pp 1-17.

Granshaw, L. (1989b) 'Fame and fortune by means of bricks and mortar: The medical profession and specialist hospitals in Britain, 1800-1948', in L. Granshaw and R. Porter (eds) *The hospital in history*, London: Routledge, pp 199-220.

Granshaw, L. (1992) 'The rise of the modern hospital in Britain', in A. Wear (ed) *Medicine in society: Historical essays*, Cambridge: Cambridge University Press, pp 197-218.

Greene, R. (1992) 'Case management: An agenda for social work practice', in B. Vourlekis and R. Greene (eds) *Social work case management*, New York, NY: Aldine de Gruyter, pp 11-25.

Griffin, J. (1991) *Dying with dignity*, London: Office of Health Economics.

Gunaratnam, Y. (1997) 'Culture is not enough. A critique of multi-culturalism in palliative care', in D. Field, J. Hockey and N. Small (eds) *Death, gender and ethnicity*, London: Routledge, pp 166-86.

Halmos, P. (1965) *The faith of the counsellors*, London: Hutchinson.

Harris, L. (1995) Personal communication, Disability Consultant, Lisa Harris Consultancies, Melbourne.

Hart, B., Sainsbury, P., and Short, S. (1998) 'Whose dying? A sociological critique of the "'good death'"', *Mortality*, vol 3, no 1, pp 65-77.

Haven Hospice (2006) Haven Hospice, Gainesville, Florida, accessed 15 November (www.havenhospice.org/htm/donations_walkway.htm).

Heal, L., Sigelman, C. and Switzky, H. (1980) 'Research on community residential alternatives for the mentally retarded', in R. Flynn and K. Nitsch (eds) *Normalization, social integration, and community services*, Baltimore, MD: University Park Press, pp 215-58.

Henderson, J. (1989) 'The hospitals of late-medieval and Renaissance Florence: A preliminary survey', in L. Granshaw and R. Porter (eds) *The hospital in history*, London: Routledge, pp 63-92.

Herlihy, D. (1995) *Women, family and society in medieval Europe: Historical essays, 1978-1991*, Providence, RI: Berghahn Books.

Higginson, I. (1996) 'Clinical audit, evaluations and outcomes', in R. Fisher and P. McDaid (eds) *Palliative day care*, London: Edward Arnold, pp 108-17.

Hill, D. and Penso, D. (1995) 'Opening doors: Improving access to hospice and specialist care services by members of black and ethnic minority communities', *Occasional Paper* 7, London: National Council for Hospice and Specialist Palliative Care Services.

Hinohara, S. (2000) 'Medicine and religion – spiritual dimension of health care', *Humane Medicine, A Journal of the Art and Science of Medicine*, accessed 27 June 2006 (www.humanehealthcare.com/Article.asp?art_id=679).

Hockley, J. and Mowatt, M. (1996) 'Rehabilitation', in R. Fisher and P. McDaid (eds) *Palliative day care*, London: Edward Arnold, pp 13-21.

Hollis, E. and Taylor, A. (1951) *Social work education in the United States: The report of a study made for the National Council on Social Work Education*, New York, NY: Columbia University Press.

Honeybun, J., Johnston, M. and Tookman, A. (1992) 'The impact of a death on fellow hospice patients', *British Journal of Medical Psychology*, vol 65, no 1, pp 67-72.

Hospice Association of America (2002) 'Hospice facts and statistics', Table 1, accessed 10 July 2006 (www.nahc.org/Consumer/hpcstats.html).

Hospice of the Florida Suncoast (2006) Clearwater, Florida, accessed 29 June (www.thehospice.org/comicrelief.htm).

Houlbrooke, R. (1998) *Death, religion and the family in England 1480-1750*, Oxford: Clarendon Press.

House, N. (1993) 'Helping to reach an understanding: Palliative care for people from ethnic minority groups', *Professional Nurse*, vol 8, no 5, pp 329-32.

House of Commons Social Services Committee (1990) *5th Report, Session 1989-90, Community care: carers*, London: HMSO.

Howe, S. (1976) 'On the causes of idiocy', in M. Rosen, G. Clark and M. Kivitz (eds) *The history of mental retardation, vol 1*, Baltimore, MD: University Park Press, pp 31-60.

Hunt, R. (1997) 'Place of death of cancer patients: Choice versus constraint', *Progress in Palliative Care*, vol 5, no 6, pp 238-42.

Ida, E., Miyachi, M., Uemura, M., Osakama, M. and Tajitsu, T. (2002) 'Current status of hospice cancer deaths both in-unit and at home (1995-2000), and prospects of home care services in Japan', *Palliative Medicine*, vol 16, no 3, pp 179–84.

Illich, I. (1976) *Limits to medicine: Medical nemesis: The expropriation of health*, London: Marion Boyars.

Illich, I. (ed) (1977) *Disabling professions*, London: Marion Boyars.

James, N. and Field, D. (1992) 'The routinization of hospice: Charisma and bureaucratization', *Social Science and Medicine*, vol 34, no 12, pp 1363-75.

Jameton, A. (1992) 'Nursing ethics and the moral situation of the nurse', in E. Friedman (ed) *Choices and conflict*, Chicago, IL: American Hospital Publishing, pp 101-9.

Jewson, N. (1976) 'The disappearance of the sick man from medical cosmology 1770-1870', *Sociology*, vol 10, no 2, pp 225-44.

JNCS (Jay Nolan Community Services) (2006) Los Angeles, accessed 20 June (www.jaynolan.org/about_us.asp).

Johnson, K. and Traustadóttir, R. (eds) (2005) *Deinstitutionalization and people with intellectual disabilities: In and out of institutions*, London: Jessica Kingsley Publishers.

Johnson, M. and Webb, C. (1995) 'Rediscovering unpopular patients: The concept of social judgement', *Journal of Advanced Nursing*, vol 21, no 3, pp 466-75.

Kalish, R. (1965) 'The aged and the dying process: the inevitable decisions', *Journal of Social Issues*, vol 21, no 4, pp 87-96.

Kane, R., Kane, R. and Ladd, R. (1998) *The heart of long-term care*, New York, NY: Oxford University Press.

Kanitsaki, O. (1998) 'Palliative care and cultural diversity', in J. Parker and S. Aranda (eds) *Palliative care: Explorations and challenges*, Sydney: MacLennan and Petty, pp 32-45.

Kaufmann, W. (1976) *Existentialism, religion and death: Thirteen essays*, New York, NY: Meridian Books.

Kearl, M. (1989) *Endings: A sociology of death and dying*, New York, NY: Oxford University Press.

Kellehear, A. (1984) 'Are we a "death-denying" society? A sociological review', *Social Science and Medicine*, vol 18, no 9, pp 713-23.

Kellehear, A. (1990) *Dying of cancer: The final year of life*, Chur: Harwood Academic Publishers.

Kellehear, A. (1998) *What is health promoting palliative care?*, Monograph, Melbourne: Palliative Care Unit, La Trobe University.

Kellehear, A. (1999) *Health promoting palliative care*, Melbourne: Oxford University Press.

Kellehear, A. (2005a) *Compassionate cities: Public health and end-of-life care*, London: Routledge.

Kellehear, A. (2005b) 'Dying in Japan', *Centre of Pacific and American Studies Newsletter*, vol 5, no 2, p 13.

Kelly, M. and May, D. (1982) 'Good and bad patients: A review of the literature and a theoretical critique', *Journal of Advanced Nursing*, vol 7, no 2, pp 147-56.

Komesaroff, P., Moss, C. and Fox, R. (1989) 'Patients' socioeconomic background: Influence on selection of inpatient or domiciliary hospice terminal care programmes', *Medical Journal of Australia*, vol 151, pp 199-201.

Krampitz, S. (1987) 'Nursing power, nursing politics', in C. Maggs (ed) *Nursing history: The state of the art*, London: Croom Helm, pp 88-106.

Kristiansen, K., Soder, M. and Tossebro, J. (1999) 'Social integration in the welfare state: Research from Norway and Sweden', in R. Flynn and R. Lemay (eds) *A quarter century of normalization and Social Role Valorization: Evolution and impact*, Ottawa: University of Ottawa Press, pp 411-24.

Kubler-Ross, E. (1975) *Death: The final stage of growth*, Englewood Cliffs, NJ: Prentice Hall.

Kugel, R. and Wolfensberger, W. (eds) (1969) *Changing patterns in residential services for the mentally retarded*, Washington, DC: President's Committee on Mental Retardation, US Government Printing Office.

Kuhn, T. (1962) *The structure of scientific revolutions*, Chicago, IL: University of Chicago Press.

Kuhse, H. (1997) *Caring: Nurses, women and ethics*, Oxford: Blackwell.

Laing, R. (1965) *The divided self: An existential study in sanity and madness*, Harmondsworth: Penguin.

Laski, F. (1980) 'Right to services in the community', in R. Flynn and K. Nitsch (eds) *Normalization, social integration, and community services*, Baltimore, MD: University Park Press, pp 167-75.

Lawton, J. (1998) 'Contemporary hospice care: The sequestration of the unbounded body and "dirty dying"', *Sociology of Health and Illness*, vol 20, no 2, pp 121-43.

Lee, D., Mackenzie, A., Dudley-Brown, S. and Chin, T. (1998) 'Case management: A review of definitions and practices', *Journal of Advanced Nursing*, vol 7, no 5, pp 933-9.

Lewis, J. (1992) 'Providers, consumers, the state and the delivery of health care services in twentieth century Britain', in A. Wear (ed) *Medicine in society: Historical essays*, Cambridge: Cambridge University Press, pp 317-46.

Lineback, L. (1987) 'A history of the Visiting Nursing Association of Greater Kansas City: The first 75 years', in C. Maggs (ed) *Nursing history: The state of the art*, London: Croom Helm, pp 124-42.

Lippman, A. (2003) 'Eugenics and public health', *American Journal of Public Health*, vol 93, no 1, p 11.

Lofland, L. (1978) *The craft of dying: The modern face of death*, Beverly Hills, CA: Sage Publications.

Lord, J. and Hutchison, P. (2003) 'Individualised support and funding: Building blocks for capacity building and inclusion', *Disability and Society*, vol 18, no 1, pp 71-86.

Loudon, I. (1992) 'Medical practitioners 1750-1850 and the period of medical reform in Britain', in A. Wear Andrew (ed) *Medicine in society: Historical essays*, Cambridge: Cambridge University Press, pp 219-48.

Lunt, B. and Hillier, R. (1981) 'Terminal care: Present services and future priorities', *British Medical Journal*, vol 283, no 6291, pp 595-98.

Lutfiyya, Z. (2003) Personal communication, Canadian Institutes of Health Research, Ottawa (www.hsf.ca/research/competition/FundInitiatives/Palliative.html).

Lynn, P. and Smith, J. (1992) *The 1991 national survey of voluntary activity in the UK,* Berkhamstead: Volunteer Centre, UK.

McEnhill, L. (2004) 'Disability', in D. Oliviere and B. Monroe (eds) *Death, dying and social differences*, Oxford: Oxford University Press, pp 97-118.

McKnight, J. (1977) 'Professionalized service and disabling help', in I. Illich (ed) *Disabling professions*, London: Marion Boyars, pp 69-91.

McKnight, J. (1995) *The careless society: Community and its counterfeits*, New York, NY: Basic Books.

Macdonald, E. and Macdonald, J. (1992) 'How do local doctors react to a hospice?', *Health Bulletin Edinburgh*, vol 50, no 5, pp 351-55.

MacIntyre, A. (1985) *After virtue*, London: Duckworth.

Macomb-Oakland Regional Center (2006) Detroit, Michigan, accessed 16 November (www.morcinc.org/about/history.htm).

Maddocks, I. (1990) 'Changing concepts in palliative care', *The Medical Journal of Australia*, vol 152, no 10, pp 535-9.

Maggs, C. (1987) 'Nursing history: Contemporary practice and contemporary concerns', in C. Maggs (ed) *Nursing history: The state of the art*, London: Croom Helm, pp 1-8.

Martin, J. (1991) 'Issues in the current treatment of hospice patients with HIV disease', in M. Amenta and C. Tehan (eds) *AIDS and the hospice community*, New York, NY: Harrington Press, pp 31-40.

Mellor, P. (1993) 'Death in high modernity: The contemporary presence and absence of death', in D. Clark (ed) *The sociology of death: Theory, culture and practice*, Oxford: Blackwell, pp 11-30.

Miller, J. and Abbott, J. (1991) 'The Connecticut Hospice Inc', in J. Miller (ed) *Community-based long term care: Innovative models*, Newbury Park, CA: Sage Publications, pp 155-73.

Miller, J. and Lombardi, T. (Jr) (1991) 'The nursing home without walls', in J. Miller (ed) *Community-based long term care: Innovative models*, Newbury Park, CA: Sage Publications, pp 138-54.

Moller, D. (1996) *Confronting death: Values, institutions and human mortality*, New York, NY: Oxford University Press.

Mor, V. and Hiris, J. (1983) 'Determinants of site of death among hospice cancer patients', *Journal of Health and Social Behavior*, vol 24, no 4, pp 375-85.

Mor, V. and Masterson-Allen, S. (1987) *Hospice care systems: Structure, process, cost and outcome*, New York, NY: Springer.

More, P. and Mandell, S. (1997) *Case management: An evolving practice*, New York, NY: McGraw-Hill.

Morgan, S. (1987) *My place*, Fremantle: Fremantle Arts Centre Press.

Murphy, C. (1989) 'From Friedenheim to hospice: A century of cancer hospitals', in L. Granshaw and R. Porter (eds) *The hospital in history*, London: Routledge, pp 221-41.

Navarro, V. (1976) *Medicine under capitalism*, New York, NY: Neale Watson Academic Publications.

Naysmith, A. (1999) 'Wider implications', in N. Bosanquet and C. Salisbury (eds) *Providing a palliative care service: Towards an evidence base*, Oxford: Oxford University Press, pp 163-72.

Neale, B. (1993) 'Informal care and community care', in D. Clark (ed) *The future for palliative care: issues of policy and practice*, Buckingham: Open University Press, pp 52-67.

Neale, B. and Clark, D. (1992) 'Informal palliative care: A review of research on needs and services', *Journal of Cancer Care*, vol 1, pp 193-98.

Newell, M. (1996) *Using nursing case management to improve health outcomes*, Gaithersburg, MD: Aspen Publishers.

Nirje, B. (1969) 'The normalisation principle and its human management implications', in R. Kugel and W. Wolfensberger (eds) *Changing patterns in residential services for the mentally retarded*, Washington, DC: Presidential Committee on Mental Retardation.

Norman, A. (1985) 'Applying theory to practice. The impact of organizational structure on programs and providers', in M. Weil, J. Karls and Associates (eds) *Case management in human service practice*, San Francisco: Jossey-Bass, pp 72-93.

North, M. (1972) *The secular priests*, London: Allen and Unwin.

Nutton, V. (1992) 'Healers in the medical marketplace: Towards a social history of Graeco-Roman medicine', in A. Wear (ed) *Medicine in society: Historical essays*, Cambridge: Cambridge University Press, pp 15-58.

O'Connor, P. (1995) 'Dying in hospital', in I. Corless, B. Germino and M. Pittman (eds) *A challenge for living: Dying, death, and bereavement*, Boston, MA: Jones and Bartlett, pp 53-67.

Office of the Public Advocate and Headway (1992) *Case management: A better approach to service delivery for people with disabilities*, Melbourne: Office of the Public Advocate.

O'Gorman, B. and O'Brien, T. (1990) 'Motor neurone disease', in C. Saunders (ed) *Hospice and palliative care: An interdisciplinary approach*, London: Edward Arnold, pp 41-5.

Olbrisch, M. and Levenson, J. (1991) 'Psychosocial evaluation of cardiac transplant candidates: An international survey of process, criteria and outcomes', *Journal of Heart and Lung Transplantation*, vol 10, pp 948-55.

O'Leary, M. (1988) *Till the shades lengthen: Caritas Christi Hospice, Kew, 1938-1988*, Melbourne: Dimond Press.

OPZ Geel (2006) 'Openbaar Psychiatrisch Ziekenhuis (OPZ) – Geel, History', accessed 29 September (www.opzgeel.be/en/algemeen/htm/history.asp).

Order of Malta (1992) *The Australian association of the Sovereign Military Order of Malta: Membership and statutes*, Melbourne: The Sovereign Military Hospitaller Order of St John of Jerusalem, of Rhodes and of Malta.

Orme, N. and Webster, M. (1995) *The English hospital 1070-1570*, New Haven, CT: Yale University Press.

Osburn, J. (1998) 'An overview of Social Role Valorization theory', *The International Social Role Valorization Journal/La revue internationale de la valorisation des roles sociaux*, vol 3, no 1, pp 7-12.

Paradis, L. and Cummings, S. (1986) 'The evolution of hospice in America: Toward organisational homogeneity', *Journal of Health and Social Behaviour*, vol 27, December, pp 370-86.

Park, K. (1992) 'Medicine and society in medieval Europe 500-1500', in A. Wear (ed) *Medicine in society: Historical essays*, Cambridge: Cambridge University Press, pp 59-90.

Parliament of Australia (1991) *Disability Services Act (1991)*, Canberra: Commonwealth Government Printer.

Parry, J. (1989) *Social work theory and practice with the terminally ill*, London: Haworth Press.

Parry-Jones, W. (1972) *The trade in lunacy: A study of private madhouses in England in the eighteenth and nineteenth centuries*, London: Routledge and Kegan Paul.

Parsons, C. (1998) 'Dying of AIDS in Australia', in J. Parker and S. Aranda (eds) *Palliative care: Explorations and challenges*, Sydney: MacLennan and Petty, pp 259-72.

Parsons, M. (2004) 'A short explanation of the Poor Law in respect of rural communities 1601-1834', accessed 16 November 2006 (www.mdlp.co.uk/resources/general/poor_law.htm).

PAT (Pets As Therapy) (2003) Reading, accessed 20 July (www.petsastherapy.org/).

'Patch Adams' (1998) Motion picture, Universal Pictures, Universal City, California, starring Robin Williams.

PAWS (Pets Are Wonderful Support) (2003) San Francisco, California, accessed 23 July (www.pawssf.org/).

Pearson, P. (1995) 'Client views of health visiting', in B. Heyman (ed) *Researching user perspectives on community health care,* London: Chapman and Hall, pp 106-20.

Pernick, M. (1997) 'Eugenics and public health in American history', *American Journal of Public Health,* vol 87, no 11, pp 1767-72.

Pernick, M. (2002) 'Taking better baby contests seriously', *American Journal of Public Health,* vol 92, no 5, pp 707-8.

Pernick, M. (2003) 'Pernick responds', *American Journal of Public Health,* vol 93, no 1, p 11.

Perrin, B. and Nirje, B. (1985) 'Setting the record straight: A critique of some frequent misconceptions of the Normalization principle', *Australian and New Zealand Journal of Developmental Disabilities,* vol 11, no 2, pp 69-74.

Perske, R. (1972) 'The dignity of risk', in W. Wolfensberger *The principle of normalization in human services,* Toronto: National Institute on Mental Retardation, pp 194-200.

Porter, R. (1989) 'The gift relation: Philanthropy and provincial hospitals in eighteenth century England', in L. Granshaw and R. Porter (eds) *The hospital in history,* London: Routledge, pp 149-78.

Porter, R. (1992a) 'Madness and its institutions', in A. Wear (ed) *Medicine in society: Historical essays,* Cambridge: Cambridge University Press, pp 277-302.

Porter, R. (1992b) 'The patient in England c1660-c1800', in A. Wear (ed) *Medicine in society: Historical essays,* Cambridge: Cambridge University Press, pp 91-118.

Porter, R. (2002) *Madness: A brief history,* Oxford: Oxford University Press.

Pridmore, A. (2006) 'Disability activism, independent living and direct payments', British Council of Disabled People, accessed 5 July (www.leeds.ac.uk/disability-studies/archiveuk/pridmore/direct%20payments%20conference%20paper%2011.pdf).

Prince and Princess of Wales Hospice (2003) Glasgow, accessed 20 July (www.ppwh.org.uk/daycarecentre.asp).

Prince and Princess of Wales Hospice (2006) Glasgow, accessed 25 July (www.ppwh.org.uk/index.cfm/page/47).

Prior, D. (1999a) 'Culturally appropriate palliative care for indigenous Australian people', in S. Aranda and M. O'Connor (eds) *Palliative care nursing: A guide to practice*, Melbourne: AUSMED Publications, pp 102-15.

Prior, D. (1999b) 'Palliative care in marginalised communities', *Progress in Palliative Care*, vol 7, no 2, pp 109-15.

Prior, L. (1989) *The social organisation of death: Medical discourse and social practices in Belfast*, Basingstoke: Macmillan.

Provencal, G. (1987) *Characteristics of a successful community living program and support service*, Melbourne: Yungaburra Foundation.

Race, D. (1999) *Social Role Valorization and the English experience*, London: Whiting and Birch.

Race, D. (2003) *Leadership and change in human services: Selected readings from Wolf Wolfensberger*, London: Routledge.

Race, D. (2004) 'Valuing people and valorization: Influences and differences between UK government policy and SRV', *International Journal of Disability, Community and Rehabilitation*, vol 3, no 1, accessed 23 June 2006 (www.ijdcr.ca/VOL03_01_CAN/articles/race.shtml).

Raetzman, S. and Joseph, S. (1999) *Long-term care in New York: Innovations in care for elderly and disabled people*, New York, NY: The Commonwealth Fund.

Ramsey, M. (1988) *Professional and popular medicine in France, 1770-1830: The social world of medical practice*, Cambridge: Cambridge University Press.

Randall, F. and Downie, R. (1999) *Palliative care ethics: A companion for all specialties* (2nd edn), Oxford: Oxford University Press.

Relf, M. and Couldrick, A. (1988) 'Bereavement support – the relationship between professionals and volunteers', in A. Gilmore and S. Gilmore (eds) *A safer death: Multidisciplinary aspects of terminal care*, New York, NY: Plenum Press, pp 133-7.

Riches, G. and Dawson, P. (2000) *An intimate loneliness: Supporting bereaved parents and siblings*, Buckingham: Open University Press.

Ritter-Teitel, J. (1996) 'New challenges and opportunities in integrated health care systems', in D. Flarey and S. Blancett (eds) *Handbook of nursing case management: Health care delivery in a world of managed care*, Gaithersburg, MD: Aspen Publishers, pp 46-67.

Robbins, M. (1998) *Evaluating palliative care: Establishing the evidence base*, Oxford: Oxford University Press.

Rosen, G. (1963) 'Historical sociology of a community institution', in E. Freidson (ed) *The hospital in modern society*, New York, NY: Free Press of Glencoe, pp 1-36.

Rosen, M., Clark, G. and Kivitz, M. (1976) 'Introduction', in M. Rosen, G. Clark and M. Kivitz (eds) *The history of mental retardation: Collected papers, vol 1*, Baltimore, MD: University Park Press, pp xiii-xxiv.

Rouget, D. and Harris, L. (1994) 'Challenging history: Empowerment through consumer participation', *Interaction*, vol 8, no 1, pp 10-14.

Rubin, A. (1992) 'Case management', in S. Rose (ed) *Case management and social work practice*, New York, NY: Longman, pp 5-20.

Rubin, M. (1989) 'Development and change in English hospitals, 1100-1500', in L. Granshaw and R. Porter (eds) *The hospital in history*, London: Routledge, pp 41-59.

Rumbold, B. (1998) 'Implications of mainstreaming hospice into palliative care systems', in J. Parker and S. Aranda (eds) *Palliative care: Explorations and challenges*, Sydney: MacLennan and Petty, pp 11-24.

Rumbold, B. (1999) 'Traditional hospice ideals and health promoting palliative care: What's new, what's not?', in M. Box and A. Kellehear (eds) *Sink or swim – Palliative care in the mainstream? Proceedings of the inaugural Victorian state conference on palliative care, Feb 10-12 1999*, Melbourne: La Trobe University, pp 63-6.

Russon, L. (1998) 'The implications of informed consent in palliative care', *European Journal of Palliative Care*, vol 4, no 1, pp 29-31.

Salisbury, C. (1997) 'What models of palliative care services have been proposed or developed in the UK, Europe, North America and Australia?', in N. Bosanquet, E. Kilberry, C. Salisbury, P. Franks, S. Kite, M. Lorentzon et al, *Appropriate and cost-effective models of service delivery in palliative care*, London: Department of Primary Health Care and General Practice, Imperial School of Medicine at St Mary's.

Sanderson, H., Kennedy, L. and Ritchie, P. (1997) *Peoples, plans and possibilities: Exploring person centred planning*, Edinburgh: SHS Trust.

Saunders, C. (1977) 'Dying they live: St Christopher's hospice', in H. Feifel (ed) *New meanings of death*, New York, NY: McGraw-Hill, pp 153-79.

Saunders, C. (1986) 'The modern hospice', in F. Wald (ed) *In quest of the spiritual component of care for the terminally ill*, New Haven, CT: Yale University School of Nursing, p 42.

Saunders, C. (1995) 'Foreword', in I. Corless, B. Germino and M. Pittman (eds) *A challenge for living: Dying, death, and bereavement*, Boston, MA: Jones and Bartlett, pp vi-ix.

Saunders, C. (1996) 'Hospice', *Mortality*, vol 1, no 3, pp 317-22.

Saunders, C. and Baines, M. (1983) *Living with dying: The management of terminal disease* (2nd edn), Oxford: Oxford Medical Publications.

Saunders, C., Summers, D. and Teller, N. (1981) *Hospice: The living idea*, Leeds: Edwin Arnold.

Schmoll, B. and Dixon, C. (1996) 'Hospice care settings', in D. Sheehan and W. Forman (eds) *Hospice and palliative care: Concepts and practice*, Sudbury: Jones and Bartlett, pp 51-9.

Scitovsky, A. (1984) '"The high cost of dying": What do the data show?', *Health and Society*, vol 62, no 4, pp 591-608.

Seale, C. (1990) 'Caring for people who die: The experience of family and friends', *Ageing and Society*, vol 10, no 4, pp 413-28.

Seale, C. (1998) *Constructing death: The sociology of dying and bereavement*, Cambridge: Cambridge University Press.

Seale, C. and Addington-Hall, J. (1994) 'Euthanasia: Why people want to die earlier', *Social Science and Medicine*, vol 39, no 5, pp 647-54.

Seale, C. and Addington-Hall, J. (1995) 'Euthanasia: The role of good care', *Social Science and Medicine*, vol 40, no 5, pp 581-7.

Seale, C., Addington-Hall, J. and McCarthy, M. (1997) 'Awareness of dying: Prevalence, causes and consequences', *Social Science and Medicine*, vol 45, no 3, pp 477-84.

Seidler, E. (1989) 'An historical survey of children's hospitals', in L. Granshaw, and R. Porter (eds) *The hospital in history*, London: Routledge, pp 181-97.

Simpson, M. (1979) *The facts of death*, New Jersey: Prentice-Hall.

Smaje, C. and Field, D. (1997) 'Absent minorities? Ethnicity and the use of palliative care services', in D. Field, J. Hockey and N. Small (eds) *Death, gender and ethnicity*, London: Routledge, pp 142-65.

Small, N. and Rhodes, P. (2000) *Too ill to talk? User involvement and palliative care*, London: Routledge.

Smith, A. (1984) 'Problems of hospices', *British Medical Journal*, vol 288, no 6425, pp 1178-9.

Smith, W. (1994) 'Building a hospice: A personal viewpoint', in W. Kornblum and C. Smith (eds) *The healing experience: Readings on the social context of health care*, Englewood Cliffs, NJ: Prentice Hall, pp 203-8.

Southeast Hospice (2006) Southeast Missouri Hospital, Cape Girardeau, Missouri, accessed 15 November (www.southeastmissourihospital.com/cancer/hospice.htm).

Spooner, D. (1996) 'Planning and development', in R. Fisher and P. McDaid (eds) *Palliative day care*, London: Edward Arnold, pp 63-82.

St Christopher's Hospice (2003a) London, accessed 23 July (www.stchristophers.org.uk).

St Christopher's Hospice (2003b) London, accessed 23 July (www.stchristophers.org.uk/page.cfm/Link=7/GoSection=6).

Stevens, J., McFarlane, J. and Stirling, K. (2000) 'Ageing and dying', in A. Kellehear (ed) *Death and dying in Australia*, Melbourne: Oxford University Press, pp 173-89.

Storey, L. (2005) 'Preferred place of care = preferred priorities for care at the end of life', Paper presented to the Annual Conference, Hospice at Home, The National Forum for Hospice at Home (UK), accessed 10 July 2006 (www.hospiceathome.org.uk/files/ppc-update-june-2005.ppt#262,12, Why do patients not die in their Place of Choice?).

Strauss, A. (1994) 'Chronic illness, the health care system, AIDS and dying', in I. Corless, B. Germino and M. Pittman (eds) *Death, dying and bereavement: Theoretical perspectives and other ways of knowing*, Boston, MA: Jones and Bartlett, pp 15-29.

Street, A. (1995) *Nursing replay: Researching nursing culture together*, Melbourne: Church Livingstone.

Street, A. (1998) 'Competing discourses within palliative care', in J. Parker and S. Aranda (eds) *Palliative care: Explorations and challenges*, Sydney: MacLennan and Petty, pp 68-81.

Street, A. and Kissane, D. (1998) 'Forecasting the future', in J. Ramadge (ed) *Australian nursing practice and palliative care: Its origins, evolution and future*, Canberra: Royal College of Nursing, pp 79-91.

Sudnow, D. (1967) *Passing on: The social organisation of dying*, Englewood Cliffs, NJ: Prentice Hall.

Szasz, T. (1961) *The myth of mental illness*, New York, NY: Holber-Harper.

Szasz, T. (1994) *Cruel compassion: Psychiatric control of society's unwanted*, New York, NY: Wiley.

Taylor, S. (2005) 'The institutions are dying, but are not dead yet', in K. Johnson and R. Traustadóttir (eds) *Deinstitutionalization and people with intellectual disabilities: In and out of institutions*, London: Jessica Kingsley Publishers, pp 93-107.

Tehan, C. (1991) 'The cost of caring for patients with HIV infection in hospice', in M. Amenta and C. Tehan (eds) *AIDS and the hospice community*, New York, NY: Haworth Press, pp 41-59.

Thompson, N. (ed) (2002) *Loss and grief: A guide for human service practitioners*, Basingstoke: Palgrave.

Thompson, N. and Thompson, S. (2005) *Community care*, Lyme Regis: Russell House Publishing.

Tigges, K. (1993) 'Quality of life: Reality or rhetoric', *Loss and Grief Care*, vol 7, no 1/2, pp 157-67.

Tronto, J. (1993) *Moral boundaries: A political argument for an ethic of care*, New York: Routledge.

Turner, V. (1969) *The ritual process*, London: Routledge & Kegan Paul.

Valins, M., Sovich, R. and Scott, G. (1996) 'The in-patient hospice: Theory and case study', in M. Valins and D. Salter (eds) *Futurecare: New directions in planning health care environments*, Oxford: Blackwell Science, pp 104-13.

van Bommel, H. (2003) Personal communication, Co-Executive Director, Legacies Inc, Ontario, accessed 2 July 2006 (www.legacies.ca/).

Very Special Kids (2003) Melbourne, accessed 20 July (www.vsk.org.au/).

Waddington, I. (1973) 'The role of the hospital in the development of modern medicine: A sociological analysis', *Sociology*, vol 7, no 2, pp 211-24.

Waddington, I. (1977) 'General practitioners and consultants in early nineteenth century England: The sociology of an intra-professional conflict', in J. Woodward and D. Richards (eds) *Health care and popular medicine in nineteenth century England: Essays in the social history of medicine*, London: Croom Helm, pp 164-88.

Walter, T. (1991) 'Modern death: Taboo or not taboo', *Sociology*, vol 25, no 2, pp 293-310.

Walter, T. (1994) *The revival of death*, London: Routledge.

Wear, A. (1992) 'Making sense of health and the environment in early modern England', in A. Wear (ed) *Medicine in society: Historical essays*, Cambridge: Cambridge University Press, pp 119-48.

Wellard, S. (1996) 'Family connections? Exploring nursing roles with families in home-based care', *Nursing Inquiry*, vol 3, no 1, pp 57-8.

West, T. (1990) 'Multidisciplinary working', in C. Saunders (ed) *Hospice and palliative care: An interdisciplinary approach*, London: Edward Arnold, pp 3-13.

Wilkinson, E. (1999a) 'Patient and carer satisfaction', in N. Bosanquet and C. Salisbury (eds) *Providing a palliative care service: Towards an evidence base*, Oxford: Oxford University Press, pp 97-130.

Wilkinson, E. (1999b) 'Problems of conducting research in palliative care', in N. Bosanquet and C. Salisbury (eds) *Providing a palliative care service: Towards an evidence base*, Oxford: Oxford University Press, pp 22-9.

Williams, P. (2004) 'Incorporating Social Role Valorisation into other contexts of needs assessment, anti-oppressive practice and the application of values', *International Journal of Disability, Community and Rehabilitation*, vol 3, no 1, accessed 23 June 2006 (www.ijdcr.ca/VOL03_01_CAN/articles/williams.shtml).

Wolfensberger, W. (1972) *The principle of normalization in human services*, Toronto: National Institute on Mental Retardation.

Wolfensberger, W. (1975) *The origin and nature of our institutional models*, New York, NY: Human Policy Press.

Wolfensberger, W. (1976a) '"Will there always be an institution?": I: The impact of epidemiological trends', in M. Rosen, G. Clark and M. Kivitz (eds) *The history of mental retardation: Collected papers, vol 2*, Baltimore, MD: University Park Press, pp 400-14.

Wolfensberger, W. (1976b) '"Will there always be an institution?": II: The impact of new service models', in M. Rosen, G. Clark and M. Kivitz (eds) *The history of mental retardation: Collected papers, vol 2*, Baltimore, MD: University Park Press, pp 415-32.

Wolfensberger, W. (1980) 'The definition of normalisation: Update, problems: Disagreements and misunderstandings', in R. Flynn and K. Nitsch (eds) *Normalization, social integration, and community services*, Baltimore, MD: University Park Press, pp 71-115.

Wolfensberger, W. (1983) 'Social Role Valorization: A proposed new term for the principle of normalization', *Mental Retardation*, vol 21, no 6, pp 234-39.

Wolfensberger, W. (1984) 'Reflections on Gibson's article', *Mental Retardation*, vol 22, no 4, pp 166-8.

Wolfensberger, W. (1992a) *The new genocide of handicapped and afflicted people* (2nd rev edn), Syracuse, NY: Author.

Wolfensberger, W. (1992b) *A guideline on protecting the health and lives of patients in hospitals, especially if the patient is a member of a societally devalued class*, Syracuse, NY: Training Institute for Human Service Planning, Leadership and Change Agentry, Syracuse University.

Wolfensberger, W. (1995) 'The SRV training package', Unpublished manuscript.

Wolfensberger, W. (1998) *A brief introduction to Social Role Valorization: A high-order concept for addressing the plight of societally devalued people, and for structuring human services* (3rd edn), Syracuse, NY: Training Institute for Human Service Planning, Leadership and Change Agentry, Syracuse University.

Wolfensberger, W. (1999) 'Response to Professor Michael Oliver', in R. Flynn and R. Lemay (eds) *A quarter century of normalization and Social Role Valorization: Evolution and impact*, Ottawa: University of Ottawa Press, pp 175-80.

Wolfensberger, W. (2002) 'Social role valorization and, or versus, "empowerment"', *Mental Retardation*, vol 40, no 3, pp 252-8.

Wolfensberger, W. and Thomas, S. (1983) *PASSING (Program analysis of service systems' implementation of normalization goals): Normalization criteria and ratings manual* (2nd edn), Toronto: National Institute on Mental Retardation.

Wootton, B. (1963) 'The law, the doctor, and the deviant', *British Medical Journal*, vol 2, pp 197-202.

Yates, P. (1998) 'Psychosocial dimensions: Issues in clinical management', in J. Parker and S. Aranda (eds) *Palliative care: Explorations and challenges*, Sydney: MacLennan and Petty.

Ziegler, H. (1992) *Changing lives, changing communities* (2nd edn), Melbourne: Wesley Central Mission.

Zola, I. (1972) 'Medicine as an institution of social control', *Sociological Review*, vol 20, no 4, pp 487-504.

Zola, I. (1977) 'Healthism and disabling medicalization', in I. Illich (ed) *Disabling professions*, London: Marion Boyars, pp 41-67.

Zollo, J. (1999) 'The interdisciplinary palliative care team: Problems and possibilities', in S. Aranda and M. O'Connor (eds) *Palliative care nursing: A guide to practice*, Melbourne: AUSMED Publications, pp 21-35.

Index

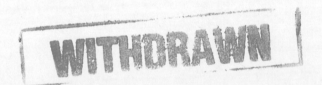